A timely book for us baby boomers who are ... ters with personal and spiritual integrity. Macgregor shares relatable stories in clear and deeply personal ways, introduces great resources for aging well, dusts off biblical sign posts to help us rediscover the kindom of God within and makes the renovating of our lives feel much less lonely. A fine resource for both personal reflection and group discussion.

—Mardi Tindal, former moderator, United Church of Canada

"Sheila Macgregor frames the discussion of retirement using images and analogies that stick. Retirement preparation is like home renovations, empty-nest vacation planning, and investment portfolio diversification. I can relate to these in my middle age. Read this book to find out how to make space for the opportunities awaiting the third-quarter of your life."

—Brad Morrison, D. Min., assistant professor of practical theology, Huron University College and author of *Already Missional: Congregations as Community Partners.*

Re-designing Your Life: A Practical Spirituality For The Second Half Of Life *is an engaging and evocative book and video study about rebuilding life after retirement. In a down-to-earth and accessible way, Sheila Macgregor offers inspiring stories from her own and others' lives and instructive input from a wide variety of authors in the field of elder studies, and wraps it all in scripture and theology that connect our story to God's story with clarity and grace. Her book is a practical and trustworthy guide to building an abundant, meaningful, and purpose-filled life after age 50. I highly recommend it for individuals and for groups.*

—Rev. Dr. Anne Beattie-Stokes, pastoral support minister, London Conference, The United Church of Canada

In a culture yearning for meaning and purpose, Sheila Macgregor offers us both. This book brings the wisdom of the ages to those of us seeking the way through the second half of our lives in compelling and practical ways. It will certainly shape the way I live my life going forward.

—Rev. Dr. Jeffrey Japinga, Executive Presbyter, Presbytery of the Twin Cities area and former Dean, Doctor of Ministry program, McCormick Theological Seminary, Chicago

Now that I have reached retirement age, I am appreciative of the adage that "aging is not for sissies." I am even more appreciative of Sheila Macgregor's thoughtful and encouraging practical spirituality for people over fifty. Full of wisdom, practical exercises, and useful suggestions, this book will help Christian women and men find meaning, satisfaction, and joy, as they enter the third and fourth stages of their lives.

—Rev. Dr. Deborah Kapp, formerly the Edward F. and Phyllis K. Campbell associate professor of urban ministry, McCormick Theological Seminary, Chicago, author of *Worship Frames: How We Shape and Interpret Our Experience of God.* (Vital Worship for Healthy Congregations)

A caring and engaging congregational minister, Sheila Macgregor has provided churches and individuals with a stimulating, personable resource that respects the many dimensions of growing older. Evocative questions open up pathways to meaningful reflection and conversation on the way to purposeful living in the second half of life. Highly recommended!

—Jane Kuepfer, MDiv PhD-c, Schlegel specialist in spirituality and aging, Conrad Grebel University, Waterloo, Ont.

Rev. Dr. Macgregor has crafted a study guide that is heartfelt, well-researched and spiritually inspired. The readers/participants become aware about the potential pitfalls and possibilities for life after fifty to engage them in preparing for the future. They are provided with practical and tangible exercises and discussion opportunities to explore both challenges and solutions in order to be able to craft and implement their own meaningful and spiritually aligned plan for the second half of life. This is a wise and worthwhile investment for anyone who wants to live a meaningful and fulfilling life after fifty and for congregations in supporting their members throughout life.

—Janet Christensen, BA, transformation maven speaker, coach, award-winning author, chief inspiration officer (& president), Dynamic Awareness Inc. Awakening Baby Boomers to pitfalls and possibilities for Life After 50.

This book is creatively written weaving together insights from theological, psychological and medical research related to aging into the mid-later years of life. The material is very engaging being presented with very helpful and thoughtful illustrations and references to the personal stories of people honestly facing the challenges and opportunities of aging. The practical suggestions gained from the authors' pastoral experience guides the reader in a very hopeful, faith informed approach to healthy aging and the life transitions we all will face in our lives.

—Paul Pearce, Centre for Healthy Aging Transitions, Carey Theological College, Vancouver.

RE-DESIGNING YOUR LIFE:
A PRACTICAL SPIRITUALITY FOR THE SECOND HALF OF LIFE

SHEILA MACDONALD MACGREGOR

*Video resources to accompany this book
are available by contacting the author at
sheila@boomerality.com*

◆ FriesenPress

Suite 300 - 990 Fort St
Victoria, BC, V8V 3K2
Canada

www.friesenpress.com

All scripture quotations are from the New Revised Standard Version of the Bible unless otherwise indicated.

ISBN
978-1-5255-1716-7 (Hardcover)
978-1-5255-1717-4 (Paperback)
978-1-5255-1718-1 (eBook)

1. RELIGION, CHRISTIAN LIFE, SPIRITUAL GROWTH

Distributed to the trade by The Ingram Book Company

For Richard —
I can't imagine spending the second half of life
with anyone other than you!

Table of Contents

Preface

Jesus said, "In my father's house are many rooms." (John 14:2) As a child, I often wondered what this house would be like. Would it be large and grand and ornate, or simple like its master? Would there be glittering Waterford crystal chandeliers in every room? Or would the light filling each room have its source in the One who is called the Light of the World?

As an adult, I understand that the house of which Jesus spoke is not made with gold and marble, or even with bricks and mortar. The house to which Jesus refers is the house that is our life, both now and in the life to come. What makes this house beautiful is not the complexity of its design, its square footage, or its polished details and lavish furnishings. What makes this house beautiful are the same things that make it a home: cozy corners in which to relax after a full day, space for learning and creativity, room for new acquaintances, cherished memories, and—most of all—the love and care of family and friends.

Today, thanks to the advances in modern medicine, the house that is our earthly life has increased in size by anywhere from twenty to thirty years. As a result, for many of us (at least in the West), there is an opportunity to redesign our lives in the second half. That's what this book is about: redesigning the house that will be our life after age fifty and beyond. The renovations we undertake may not always be easy—or even something we really wanted or planned to undertake. The walls surrounding us day in and day out may need to be repaired or knocked down completely so that we can embrace new dreams and passions. They will need to include expansive windows and wide doors that draw us out into God's world. Our renovated house must be open to welcoming others we encounter along life's path, including those who are very different from ourselves. The house that is our life cannot stop at the edge of a well-manicured lawn—otherwise, it will never become the home Christ wants to give us. Instead, it needs to sing the story of who we are as God's faithful servants.

This book was made by possible by the McGeachy Senior Scholarship awarded to me by the United Church of Canada Foundation. It had its origins in a Doctor of Ministry thesis project I undertook at McCormick Theological Seminary in Chicago. Its goal is to help people transition into the second half of life and to consider where and how God is calling them to serve in these years. My hope is that this resource can be used by church study groups or as a personal devotional. Groups may wish to avail themselves of a video resource that accompanies this study. While not exhaustive, the book study seeks to introduce readers to a number of key people working in this still relatively new field. If it does no more than spur others on to read these authors, then the project will have been successful. However, the work is also part of a deeply personal spiritual quest. As one who is now well into the second half of life and for whom formal retirement is less than a decade away, this work represents my own discernment as to where God is calling me to serve in this postmeridian period of my life. I am thankful to have your company as you join me on this spiritual quest.

Sheila Macdonald Macgregor,
January 1st, 2018,
Exeter, Ontario

Chapter 1:
Building an Atrium

"Unless the Lord builds the house,
those who build it labor in vain."
—Psalm 127:1–2

An Extra Room at the Centre of Your Life!

My friend Maralyn and her husband, Robert, live in a lovely, century-old home in a small village just outside London, Ontario. They have been there for nearly twenty-five years. They love that their house has character, with a large garden out back, and that they can commute to their jobs in the city in minutes while enjoying the more peaceful pace of life in a small rural community. It has been the ideal place to raise their three children.

Over the years, Maralyn and Robert have undertaken a number of renovations to their home. When their children were young, they finished a corner of the basement and turned it into a playroom. Like most century-old homes, the basement did not have a high ceiling, but since the children were still small, this really didn't matter. The kids loved their playroom and enjoyed having a space where they could make as much mess as they liked. Their parents enjoyed it, too. It meant that they knew where their children were and that they could have some quiet space to themselves on the main floor while the children played safely and happily downstairs.

As the children grew older—and taller—a different kind of arrangement was needed. What they really craved now was a larger, sunnier room on the main level, a room that the whole family could enjoy. Since their current living room was too small, they decided to build a bright, airy family room on the back of their home. They still planned to keep the smaller living room as a place where they could read or welcome guests, but an interesting thing happened when they added the family room: they no longer used their living room at all. Instead, they found themselves spending all their time in the family room. So they decided to convert their current living room into a bedroom for their eldest daughter. And the playroom downstairs? It has taken on other reincarnations, as a work room, a storage area, and even a small in-home gym!

You, too, may have been involved in home renovations in the past. If so, like my friends Maralyn and Robert, the first thing you may have discovered when you added a room to your house is that "add" is generally the wrong word, because the way you use all the rest of the house will be affected by the change. Indeed, even your relationships and the way you live and organize your time will change.

This is often what happens when we renovate or add an extra room to our house. Cultural anthropologist Mary Catherine Bateson describes how our lives change as we alter the spaces in which we live:

> Existing rooms begin to be used differently, sounds echo in new ways, community and privacy take on new meanings. Gaps open where familiar items have been

shifted to the new space and new acquisitions fill them. The new room is not simply "tacked on" to the east or west side of the house; it represents a new configuration of the entire building and the lives it shelters.[1]

Bateson notes that this is what longevity is like. With additional years added to our lives, new spaces open up, and new room is created, leading to changes in the way we organize our time and relationships. For example, when Canada's Old Age Pension was signed into law in May 1928, the life expectancy for a Canadian man was sixty, and for a Canadian woman, sixty-two. Now we can expect to live far longer. Demographers tell us that since the beginning of the twentieth century, many have been given another thirty years, twenty of those since World War II alone. Today, for example, when people turn fifty, most can expect thirty more years of productive life compared with previous generations. The result is that a new room has been added to the house we call life.

Bateson says, "We have not added decades to life expectancy by simply extending old age. We have opened up a new space partway through the life course—a second and different kind of adulthood that precedes old age—and, as a result, every stage of life is undergoing change."[2] What this will look like will be as varied as our individual imaginations.

In my own life, I can remember that, as a child, I would occasionally see photos in our local newspaper depicting five generations of a family. These photos were newsworthy because most people back then did not get to know their great-grandparents. Many of us did

---

1 Mary Catherine Bateson, *Composing a Further Life: The Age of Active Wisdom*, (New York, A. Knopfe, 2010), 10–11.

2 Ibid.

not even have the privilege of getting to know all our grandparents. Today, it is not uncommon for children to have a relationship with great-grandparents who are still fit and agile. My friends Betty and Al regularly babysit their grandchildren's young children. They say it's the best time of their life. When their children and grandchildren were young, they were both still working full-time. Now they get to play with their grandchildren's children!

If we are getting to play with our great-grandchildren, we are also getting to spend more time caring for our elderly parents and grandparents. I well recall, too, how my mother-in-law retired from a lengthy career in teaching to care for her elderly parents, who lived to be ninety-seven-and-a-half and 102. When they died, she was already well into her seventies. Although she continues to be healthy and active in her mid-eighties, there is no question that the longevity revolution placed some major limitations on the first fifteen years of her retirement, as she struggled to meet the care needs of her mother and father.

The important thing to remember is that the second half of life will be different for everyone. Some will need to spend more time caring for elderly parents, like my mother-in-law. Some will have the fun of looking after grandchildren and even great-grandchildren, like my friends Betty and Al. Many others will find deep satisfaction from their careers, or reinvent new careers. And others will have more time for important volunteer work—or maybe a combination of both.

To be sure, not all will retire at age sixty-five or seventy. For example, my friend Ric retired at the age of fifty-two after a successful thirty-year-teaching career. He then went on to work part-time at the college of education, where he taught an online course and supervised practice teachers.

Another friend retired from a career in the armed forces while still in his forties. While most of us can still expect to retire around the age of sixty-five, many others will work full- or part-time for far longer. My father, a lawyer, did not close his law office until he was well into his eighty-first year. Some of us, in fact, do our best work in the second half of life. For example, it is said that if Winston Churchill had died before his sixty-fifth birthday, his political career would have been considered a failure. Instead, he is remembered as the great champion who led his people—and much of the free world—through one of the most tumultuous periods in their history. In 1950, when he was seventy-six years old, *Time* magazine called him "The Man of the Twentieth Century". He would continue to serve as prime minister until 1955 when he was just eighty-one years young! Clearly, the second half of life is not a cookie-cutter process. It's different for everyone!

Supersizing the Life Span

To borrow an advertising slogan from McDonald's, we have now "supersized" the human life span. Traditionally, for example, the human pattern has followed a three-generation structure:

1. Infants, children, and those approaching adulthood (now called adolescents).

2. Adults, who work to maintain society and who produce and rear children.

3. Older adults, who are past their reproductive and child-rearing years, often in declining health.

Back in the 1980s, an historian at Cambridge University by the name of Peter Laslett realised that this pattern was changing. In the past, if people made it to retirement, most of them were frail and worn out. But in the late twentieth century, he noticed that something very different was happening. Instead of being the exception, healthy, active people in their seventies, eighties, and older had become so common that Laslett began to believe that the old three-stage model of human development no longer worked and that we needed a fresh map of life. Instead of thinking of life as falling into three main stages—childhood, adulthood, and old age— he argued that we need to think of four stages. As he noted, the healthy, active, early part of retirement wasn't very much like the frail, inactive, later part. They were altogether different ages in life.[3]

Thanks to advances in biomedicine, there has been a profound change in the human condition. We have inserted a whole new developmental stage into the life cycle, a second stage of adulthood, not an extension tacked onto old age. Laslett calls this the Third Age. Not surprisingly, Laslett was one of the founders of the University of the Third Age (U3A). Himself a fine role model of life in the Third Age, his book on this subject, *A Fresh Map of Life: The Emergence of the Third Age*, was published when he was seventy-four. Rather than being "over the hill," he argued that people in this stage could be "climbing the summit of life."[4]

The point is that now, for the first time in history, we have a four-generation society, which includes at its centre a new generation of active grandparents who are mobile and engaged. Moreover, many are keen to find ways to serve and give back to their communities. Most people in this

---

3   John E. Nelson and Richard N. Bolles, *What Colour is Your Parachute? For Retirement. Planning a Prosperous, Healthy, and Happy Future* (Berkeley: The Speed Press, 2010), 16.

4   Peter Laslett, *A Fresh Map of Life: The Emergence of the Third Age* (Cambridge: Harvard University Press, 1991).

stage of life have much wisdom to share, especially years of real on-the-job experience.

But wisdom is about much more than knowledge learned on the job. The gift of years enables us to contribute a much-needed long-term perspective when it comes to matters of social, political, and personal importance. No longer consumed with career advancement and the joys, but also the very real demands, of raising a family, we now have an opportunity to serve our communities by bringing to the table a viewpoint that is informed by years of experience and time for thoughtful reflection.

Dr. Marianne Mellinger has spent many years researching and teaching about the spirituality of aging. Until recently, she was the coordinator of the spirituality and aging program at the Schlegel-University of Waterloo Research Institute for Aging. Mellinger points to another fact that may contribute to a special kind of wisdom in our mature years. She notes that, by the time most people reach the second half of life, they will likely have experienced a number of changes in life.[5] Quoting William Willimon, she says that probably sixty-five percent of all major changes happen after the age of sixty-five. These include, among other life-changing events, the loss of a spouse, the loss of a job, and the loss of health. However our wisdom comes—and often it will be the result of wrestling with sorrow and disappointment—we have the ability to *act on it* and the responsibility to *pass it on*.

In his first Letter to the Corinthians, chapter 12, the Apostle Paul reminds us that "we are each given particular gifts of the Spirit." We are

---

5   Interview with Dr. Marianne Mellinger, July 26, 2016, Conrad Grebel College, University of Waterloo, Waterloo, Ont.

all called to serve Christ in various ways, according to our gifts. One of the ways we serve, according to the United Church of Canada *Song of Faith*, is by "build[ing] up the community of wisdom."[6] Indeed, this may well be the best way that those of us in the second half of life can live out our calling to Jesus Christ and his church.

The Keepers of Meaning

Perhaps the loveliest descriptor of people in this stage of life was coined by Harvard professor and psychiatrist George Vaillant. He calls them the "keepers of meaning."[7] They are the ones who dispense wisdom and experience to the next generation. The keepers of meaning are not simply concerned with the care of individuals, but with preserving the best of the culture's traditions and building a more just society.

Daniel Levinson would agree wholeheartedly. In his writing, Levinson argues that those in the second half of life can serve as important models, supporters, sponsors, and teachers to younger generations in the church and the wider community. Moreover, he notes that we are the ones who act as "encouragers" of the next generation by "believing in their dreams."[8]

Sadly, we often fail to appreciate the importance of the gift of encouragement. And, yet, where would most of us be without the encouragement of parents, teachers, coaches, employers, and friends who believed in us? Where would Helen Keller be without Annie Sullivan? Where

---

6   The United Church of Canada, *A Song of Faith: A Statement of Faith of the United Church of Canada, L'Église Unie du Canada*, 2006.

7   George E. Vaillant, *Aging Well: Surprising Guideposts to a Happier Life from the Landmark Harvard Study of Adult Development.* (New York: Hachette Book Group, 2002), 10.

8   Daniel J. Levinson, *The Seasons of a Man's Life* (Toronto: Ballantine Books, 1978), 99.

would Jackie Robinson be without the encouragement of his older brother Matthew, or without the faith and determination of Dodgers owner Branch Ricky? Where would famous author Maya Angelou be without her beloved teacher Mrs. Flowers? Or Oprah Winfrey without the encouragement of her Grade 4 teacher, Mrs. Duncan, who taught her "not to be afraid of being smart."[9] Encouragement plays a big role in determining a person's success in life and his or her general well-being. As such, its power should not be underestimated.

While encouragement is a gift in which all people can share, those of us who find ourselves in the second half of life are particularly well positioned to seek out and encourage those from whom special talent, virtues, and ideas may be struggling to emerge. Indeed, the gift of another twenty or thirty years means that we are uniquely placed to become their mentors and encouragers.

The bible is full of examples of encouragers who mentored younger disciples. Jethro mentored Moses. Moses mentored Joshua and the elders of Israel. Eli mentored Samuel. Samuel mentored Saul and David. Elijah mentored Elisha. Naomi mentored Ruth. Mordecai mentored Esther. Priscilla and Aquila mentored Apollos. Jesus mentored the twelve disciples. Paul mentored Titus, Timothy, and many others. Indeed, throughout the scriptures, the role of the elder as mentor and encourager is held in high regard. The elder is the bridge-builder between generations, the one who is able to help us discern our real potential.[10] The author of the Letter to the Colossians took

---

9   *Ilene Cooper, Up Close: Oprah Winfrey,* (Puffin, London, 2008), p. 33.

10   Zalman Schachter-Shalomi and Ronald S. Miller, *From Age-ing to Sage-ing. A Revolutionary Approach to Growing Older* (New York: Time-Warner Books, 1997), 58–60.

his own role as encourager very seriously. There, he writes to the community of believers at Colossae: "May you be made strong with all the strength that comes from his glorious power, and may you be prepared to endure everything with patience, while joyfully giving thanks to the Father, who has enabled you to share in the inheritance of the saints in the light" (Colossians 1:11–12).

Anishinaabe Elder Art Solomon: "It's That Simple!"

What Vaillant, Levinson, and Bateson write are things our First Nations brothers and sisters have known about and practised for centuries. The late Arthur Solomon, a spiritual elder of the Anishinaabe First Nation, once explained the role of the one who finds him or herself in the second half of life in words that mean the same thing. He said:

> You see, the elder, the concept for me is like if you go into a strange land and you don't know the country and you're swamped and there's muskegs and there's bad places to travel and there's good places to travel. So, the ones who have been there longer are the good guides because they know how to get around the swamps, know where to go on. It doesn't matter if there's a trail. They know that country. You know the channel, on the north side of the channel? That was cut by glaciers, the second to last one, and they cut deep. The last one that came down, they cut this way almost directly across the other. What they have left is all these whalebacks or humpback, and if you're travelling close to the borders of the channel on the far side, then you're always going up and down and around. Always like that. But if you go maybe a half

mile north, you're walking on good land. That's how simple it is. So, there are in fact guides who have been there who have each individually lived through their own hell and have found their way and they are in fact guides. So, if you are going into a strange land, and God knows it's strange to so many young people, and [if you] can avoid all that and ensure [yourself] a good trip, that's really what it is. It's that simple.[11]

Solomon understands how important it is to have good guides as we traverse this often strange and dangerous land we call life. United Church minister and spiritual elder of the Aamjiwnaang First Nation Rev. Matthew Stevens talks about the profound influence the elders have had on his life, especially Solomon. He writes, "There's never a day that goes by that I don't have at least a few occasions to recall a teaching Art shared with me, the most significant of which was: 'As freely as you have received these teachings, be ever ready and willing to share them just as freely with those you meet who can make good use of the guidance.'"[12]

This sounds a lot like another great teacher and guide: Jesus of Nazareth. In Matthew's Gospel, our Lord instructs his disciples: "Freely you have received; freely give" (Matthew 10:8). Jesus knew that the path to the Kingdom comes through service and by helping others along their life's path. It is as we use our gifts to support and guide and serve others that we experience the blessed life.

---

11   S. M. Stiegelbauer, *What is an Elder? What do Elders Do? First Nation Elders as Teachers in Culture-Based Urban Organizations*, Ontario Institute for Studies in Education of the University of Toronto, pp. 41–42.

12   Email Correspondence from Rev. Matthew Stevens, June 18, 2016.

Echoing Jesus's teaching was St. Paul. In his *First Letter to the Corinthians*, the Apostle Paul writes that we are "called to be servants of Christ and stewards of the mysteries of God." Paul is talking about all Christians, and in particular those who take on leadership roles in the church. But this is also the special role of all of us who have entered the second half of life. In a unique way, we are called to be stewards of the mysteries of God, stewards of the Word. It is to us to pass on our faith, our stories, and our traditions to those who follow. In many ways, we are like runners in a relay race, where the runner behind us runs by our side for a while, and then we pass on the baton of our traditions to them. We thus find ourselves in that part of the race where we are running side by side with those who are coming up behind us.

An Atrium at the Centre of Our Lives!

What a bonus these years can be! Bateson regards this extra period that many of us are given as an extra room in our house. She believes, however, that it should be thought of not so much as a room added onto the back, but as a kind of atrium in the centre of our house, with doorways to all other stages or relationships or rooms and even open to the sky. As she writes, "We have changed the shape and meaning of a lifetime in ways we do not yet fully understand."[13] Just as adding a new room to our physical house changes the way we use the other rooms, so, too, will an "extra room" in our lives have a major impact on our marriages, relationships with children and siblings, friendships, education, work, and retirement.

The metaphor of the atrium at the centre of our house seems most appropriate to the transition into the second half of life, as we search for our

---

13   Bateson, *Composing a Further Life*, 11.

next step. It is also a good biblical metaphor. For example, the scripture and many other spiritual writings often refer to our life as a kind of house, a home that we inhabit during our earthly years. Of course, Jesus also depicts the life to come as a house, a mansion with many rooms. As co-creators with God, you and I have a part to play in building this home.

If you have attended a lot of church weddings, you will know that the marriage service frequently begins with a passage of scripture from Psalm 127: "Unless the Lord builds the house, those who build it labour in vain. In all your ways acknowledge God and God will make straight your path." If we are going to be successful in our house-building, God needs to be at the centre. How we build our new room with God or navigate our new atrium is the focus of this study. To keep our focus, therefore, we will require a few ongoing spiritual practices.

First is *knowing yourself*. Knowing what gives you joy—even as that changes over time. Who are you now that you are no longer what you used to do? This is the primary question of all who enter into the second half of life, particularly as we retire. What are the things that feed you spiritually and give your life meaning? This is important. Many people come up to retirement with a good financial plan, but very few have a good plan for what they are going to do next with their time. They may say, Oh, we're going to relax, without realizing that full-time recreation isn't going to be satisfying to most of them. So, we really need a time to ask: "What is fundamental to me, and how can I have that in the years ahead?" We're going to be considering some of these things in the chapters that follow.

Another essential aspect of knowing the grace of God's spirit is *what we are willing to give away*. The practice of giving away our treasures is a lifelong spiritual one. The best-lived life is one in which we give and not just receive—the more giving, the better. While "giving away" can and does include material things, it is primarily about giving of ourselves. When we spend our lives giving love and kindness, we build a storehouse of goodwill and make this earth a home that we want to live in, a world that takes seriously the future of our grandchildren and our great-nieces and -nephews. And just as important as giving love away, we'll see, is knowing *what things we ought to leave behind.*

Another consideration is the willingness to address the difficult questions in life and the need also to remain open to surprises. For example, I love the story about the son who wanted talk to his aged and somewhat forgetful mother about what inevitably lay ahead, her death, but he was stumbling about a good deal. Finally, he said, "Mother, you're getting along in age, and who knows what may happen? I mean, shouldn't we make a few decisions about arrangements?"

The old lady kept silent, but was smiling calmly, so the son pressed on. "I mean, Mom, do you want to be buried or cremated?"

His mother patted his cheek, then replied, "Well, son, I don't know. Why don't you just surprise me?" As we move into the second half of life, our spiritual health requires several things, namely, that:

1. We come to truly know ourselves.

2. We practise generosity.

3. We develop a good sense of humour and remain open to the surprises of the spirit.

4. We choose our place in the future.

These Bonus Years Are Too Precious: Don't Leave Them to the Snake!

> *Now the serpent was more crafty than any other wild animal that the Lord God had made. He said to the woman, "Did God say, 'You shall not eat from any tree in the garden'?"* [2] *The woman said to the serpent, "We may eat of the fruit of the trees in the garden;* [3] *but God said, 'You shall not eat of the fruit of the tree that is in the middle of the garden, nor shall you touch it, or you shall die.'"* [4] *But the serpent said to the woman, "You will not die;* [5] *for God knows that when you eat of it your eyes will be opened, and you will be like God, knowing good and evil."* [6] *So when the woman saw that the tree was good for food, and that it was a delight to the eyes, and that the tree was to be desired to make one wise, she took of its fruit and ate; and she also gave some to her husband, who was with her, and he ate. 7 Then the eyes of both were opened, and they knew that they were naked; and they sewed fig leaves together and made loincloths for themselves.*
>
> *– Genesis 3:1–7*

Many ancient religions have creation myths that try to make sense of the world and its origins, as well as our place in it. Such stories have meaning because, through them, we discover who we are.

According to the creation story we find in Genesis 3:1–7, Adam and Eve are the first human beings to have inhabited the earth. In this story, they talk with God, their creator, and they understand what God wants. God tells them that they will have dominion over all the plants and animals in the Garden of Eden, but there is one tree in the centre of the garden from which God prohibits Adam and Eve from eating. However, the serpent tricks Eve into eating fruit from the forbidden tree. Consequently, God curses the serpent and the ground and punishes Adam and Eve by banishing them from the garden.

In the past, many theologians thought that the problem was that Adam and Eve disobeyed God's rule about the tree. Normally, we have seen "pride" as the real villain in this story—the fact that Adam and Eve desire to be wise like God and, indeed, to be equal in power to God.

Harvey Cox, who served as a professor at Harvard Divinity School until his retirement in 2009, sees this story differently. He wrote a wonderful book called *On Not Leaving It to the Snake*.[14] The problem, he says, wasn't that Adam and Eve disobeyed God's rule. The real problem was that they let the snake decide whether they should eat the forbidden fruit. Cox says this story is not about pride or our human attempt to be more than what we are. Rather, he says, it is more about sloth, our unwillingness to be everything we were intended to be.

The word "sloth" is not used much these days, but we know what it means. It's an ugly word, which in English has come to mean indolence or laziness. It is also the name given to an unattractive animal who likes to hang inertly from tree branches. The sloth never makes any decisions for itself. It just lets life happen to it.

Retired minister Paul C. Clayton says that this story from Genesis contains an important message for those of us entering the second half of life or that period we call retirement.[15] Too often. we suffer from the

---

14   Harvey Cox. *On Not Leaving It to the Snake* (New York: MacMillan, 1967).

15   Paul C. Clayton, *Called for Life: Finding Meaning in Retirement* (Herndon, VA: The Alban Institute, 2008), 58–60.

sin of sloth, not the sin of pride. That is, too often, we leave things to the snake! The danger as we enter this period in our lives is our inclination to let chance, rather than choice, decide how we will live the rest of our lives. By refusing to take responsibility for our future, we may miss our calling. Slothfulness is letting the snake decide what we will do with the rest of our lives. And there are lots of snakes around who would be only too happy to take the decision away from us!

In fact, the temptation to just drift into life can be an even greater challenge in the second half of life than it is in the first half. Slick advertisers with beautiful, glossy brochures that tout carefree retirement living, always with people who are exactly alike and have the very same interests, often delude their clients into believing that by purchasing one of their luxury homes they are not just buying a house, they are also purchasing a "lifestyle." But a lifestyle is a poor substitute for the life of meaning and joy that Jesus promises his followers. I wonder if Jesus did not have these slick hucksters in mind when he proclaimed, "the thief comes only to steal and kill and destroy. I came that they may have life, and have it abundantly". (John 10:10). To be sure, Jesus did not say, "I have come that you may have a lifestyle filled with endless rounds of golf and tennis and gourmet lunches by the pool." Jesus said, I have come "so that my joy may be in you and so that your joy may be complete" (John 15:11). Such joy, as the famous missionary doctor Albert Schweitzer once observed, comes with a far different kind of price tag. As he said once to a group of students graduating from university, "The only ones of you who will be truly happy in life are those who seek and find a way to serve."[16]

---

16   Mark Link, *100 Stories for Special Occasion Homilies* (Allen, TX: Tabor Publishing, 1992), 28.

The snake would tell us: let me take care of all your retirement needs. You just relax and enjoy. But how much fun and relaxation can one really handle? Retirement coach, Janet Christensen, CEO of Dynamic Awareness Inc. in London, Ontario, says she once challenged one of her pre-retirement clients to play golf every day while he was away on vacation, just as he said he was going to do in retirement. He quickly found that it wasn't all it was cracked up to be and golf began to feel just like a job.[17]

"It's not that you don't golf," she explains. "It's finding that healthy balance and for some people it can also be the new social interaction. It's about really finding the meaning and fulfillment in your life."[18]

The reality is that most people do not spend very much time preparing themselves emotionally or spiritually for retirement. As Christensen comments: "To put it in a nutshell, many people spend more time planning a two-week vacation than they do the second half of their life, the retirement stage of their life. . . . Those that do take some time to do the planning focus on the financial [aspect] and not anything else."[19] They move into retirement with no clear sense of who they are or what they are to do.

The urgent point of retirement is in the biblical creation story. Retirement is the opportunity we are given to choose our place in the future. Many of us spent years preparing for the first half of life. There were the years we spent in elementary school and high school. Then, for some, there was college or university, or maybe an apprenticeship. We invested a lot of time and energy in preparing for the first half of life. Should we not do the same

---

17   Interview with Janet Christensen, July 19, 2016, London, Ont.

18   Ibid.

19   Ibid.

for our second half of life? As famous psychoanalyst Carl Jung surmised years ago, "A human being would certainly not grow to be seventy or eighty years old if this longevity had no meaning to the species to which he belonged. The afternoon of human life must also have a significance of its own and cannot be merely a pitiful appendage to life's morning."[20] It has a purpose all its own and that purpose, as aging specialist Laura Carstensen asserts wisely, is not a thirty-year vacation and certainly "not to help developers populate Sun City with shuffleboard players."[21]

I think that the problem is that society asks too little of retirees or of those who find themselves in life's second half. The kinds of trivial pursuits with which much of the retirement industry seeks to bait people often fall woefully short of the joy God wants to give us. Over sixty years ago, psychologist Abraham Maslow noted that one of the basic behaviours of the "self-actualized" or truly fulfilled human being was the ability to take responsibility and work hard. The people who develop to their full stature are those who do the best they can and make full use of their talents and potentialities. As he wrote:

> Capacities clamor to be used, and cease their clamor only when they are well used. That is, capacities are also needs. Not only is it fun to use our capacities, but it is also necessary. The unused capacity or organ can become a disease centre or else atrophy, thus diminishing the person.[22]

---

20   Carl Jung, *Modern Man in Search of a Soul* (New York: Harcourt, Brace and World, 1933), 109.

21   Laura Carstensen, *A Long Bright Future* (New York, Public Affairs, 2011), 88.

22   A. H. Maslow, "Some Basic Propositions of Holistic-Dynamic Psychology," unpublished paper, Brandeis University, quoted in Betty Friedan, *The Feminine Mystique* (New York: W.W. Norton & Company, 2013), 381.

To cease using our capacities simply because we have retired from our day job or paid employment, Maslow argued, is to forfeit our humanity. It is through our work, whether paid or voluntary, that we find our life's purpose. About 125 years ago, the great psychologist William James said, "We measure ourselves by many standards. Our strength and our intelligence, our wealth, and even our good luck, are things that warm our heart and make us feel ourselves a match for life. But deeper than all such things, and able to suffice unto itself without them, *is the sense of the amount of effort that we can put forth*" (italics added).[23] It's interesting that the oft longed-for freedom from our day-to-day work to which so many look forward in retirement, may, in fact, be more of a curse than a blessing.

This is especially noteworthy, as many Christians still associate work with the punishment inflicted on humanity at the time of the fall. However, as Regent College Professor Emeritus Dr. R. Paul Stevens reminds us, "the command to work was given *before* the fall and hence work is meant to be a blessing, not a curse."[24] The author of the *Book of Ecclesiastes* would agree. He writes: "I know that there is nothing better for people than to be happy and to do good while they live. That each of them may eat and drink, and find satisfaction in all their toil—this is the gift of God" (Ecclesiastes 3:12–14).

In a workshop that Stevens co-leads with Dr. Paul Pearce at CHAT (Centre for Healthy Aging Transitions, Carey Theological Institute, Vancouver), he argues that a life fixated only on leisure activities denies the image of God in which we are created. Reflecting on Genesis 1:26–28, Stevens notes that God is a worker and as creatures created

---

23   William James, *Psychology* (New York: Henry Holt and Company, 1892), 458.

24   R. Paul Stevens, *Work Matters: Lessons from Scripture* (Grand Rapids: William B. Eerdmans Publishing Company, 2012), Loc. 120 of 1854.

in God's image, we are called to be workers, too. Moreover, as he continues, work is good for us. Building on the theology of holocaust martyr Dietrich Bonhoeffer, he says that work not only gets us out of ourselves, but it also gets us into the lives of others and, hence, is a practical way of loving our neighbours. Indeed, it is through work, Stevens says, that we advance the work of the Kingdom of God.[25]

What an awesome opportunity we have been given! The challenge to help build the commonwealth of God must not be taken lightly. The good news is that many of us have been handed a truly remarkable gift: possibly an extra thirty years of life. This extra room—or extra period we have been given—is a prospect that was not available to many in previous generations and even today is seldom available to many living in other parts of our world. We are standing on "holy ground." Our calling does not stop at fifty-five or sixty-five or some arbitrary retirement age. There is a whole new room at the centre of our lives, a whole new opportunity not to be wasted, and today God calls us to embrace the possibilities before us with hope, love, and joy. The second half of life can be one of the most fulfilling and rewarding periods of our lives. To quote the United Church *Song of Faith,*

> In and with God, we can direct our lives toward right relationship
> With each other and with God. . . .
> We can accept our mortality and finitude, not as a curse,
> But as a challenge to make our lives and choices matter.[26]

---

25   Interview with R. Paul Stevens, October 25, 2016, Regent College, Vancouver, BC., and in a workshop on October 29, 2016, Carey Theological College, Vancouver, BC.

26   The United Church of Canada, *A Song of Faith: A Statement of Faith of the United Church of Canada, L'Église Unie du Canada,* 2006.

So, let's not leave it to the snake! Instead, let's "make our lives and choices matter!"

For Further Reading:

Mary Catherine Bateson, *Re-Composing A Life*. (New York, A. Knopfe, 2010.)

William Bridges, *Transitions: Making Sense of Life's Changes*, 2nd Edition. (Cambridge, DaCapo Press, 2004.)

Paul C. Clayton, *Called for Life. Finding Meaning in Retirement*. (Rowman & Littlefield Publishers, 2008)

R. Paul Stevens, *Aging Matters. Finding Your Calling for the Rest of Your Life*. (Wm. B. Eerdmans Publishing Company, 2016)

For Viewing:

The Best Exotic Marigold Hotel, directed by John Madden, 2012.

Re-Designing Your Life: A Practical Spirituality for the Second Half of Life, Sheila Macdonald Macgregor, Wib Dawson, videographer and editor, 2017.

Questions for Discussion:

Watch the Introduction and Session One of the videos that have been made to accompany this book and then discuss the following. Note: if you are leading a study group, you may not have time to discuss all the questions. Choose those that you feel will be most helpful to your group.

1. **a)** You have been given unlimited resources to add a room to your house. There are no planning restrictions. Draw a rough floor plan. Don't worry about drawing things to scale. Just get out your pencil and have fun! What will this extra room be used for? Think about what you will need in this room in order for it to fulfill its purpose (books, gym equipment, telescope, art supplies, gardening tools, woodworking machinery, baking supplies). Don't forget to include windows to let the sunshine in!

    b) What does this room tell you about yourself? Are there any surprises? Consider how this room might affect the way you use the rest of your house. Take ten minutes to write down your thoughts.

2. The bible often refers to our lives as a kind of house. Jesus also depicts the life to come as a house with "many dwelling places" or rooms. If you think of the twenty to thirty extra years that many in our day are given as an extra room in your house, what does this new room look like for you? How could this room call you to service in the world?

3. *Knowing Yourself:*

a) Write down ten short responses to the question: "Who am I?" Go back over your list now and delete three items. Do this twice more. What did you learn about how you see yourself?

b) Now read Ephesians 2:10 "For we are God's masterpiece. He has created us anew in Christ Jesus, so we can do the good things he planned for us long ago" (NLT). What does this tell you about how God sees you?

c) In I Corinthians 12:4, the Apostle Paul writes: "Now there are varieties of gifts, but the same Spirit; and there are varieties of services, but the same Lord." This may be a good time to do a Spiritual Gifts Inventory. There are many good resources that can be downloaded online for free. Evangelical Lutheran Church of America has a good spiritual gifts assessment tool. A good list of such resources can also be found on the Diocese of Toronto, Anglican Church of Canada website under the heading "Gifts Discernment."

d) Start a gratitude journal. Once a day name at least three things you are grateful for in life. Do this throughout the duration of this course.

4. Read Genesis 3:1-7. Building on Harvey Cox's work, *On Not Leaving it to the Snake,* Paul Clayton argues that the temptation to let others decide who and what we will become is especially strong in the second half of life.

a) Google "retirement lifestyle." What images are used to advertise retirement living? What is the message being conveyed? Compare this with the search for "meaningful retirement" or "retirement Christian service." What do you notice? Which pictures feel more like "home" to you?

b) Do you agree with the author that retirement industries often want to sell us a retirement "lifestyle"? Contrast this to Jesus' message in John 10:10 that He "has come to give

[us] life, and to have it to the full." What is the difference between being sold a "lifestyle" and being given "a full life" in Christ? (N.B. If this is a group exercise, you may wish to take some time in your group session to flip through some magazines that contain advertisements aimed at those in the second half of life. What is the primary message about retirement that these ads seek to convey? How do they contrast with the life Christ wants to give us?)

c) What resources can you use to discern your calling and help you focus on the life Christ wants to give you?

d) Does the abundant life that Christ promises mean just for me or is it about abundant life for all? If it is for all, how does that affect the choices we make?

5. Read Genesis 1:27:

"So, God created humankind in his image,
in the image of God he created them;
male and female he created them."

Paul Stevens writes that God, who is a worker and who created us in the divine image, calls us also to be workers. "We should work until we die." (Stevens, *Aging Matters*, p. 11.) Contrast this to the contemporary advertisements that continually portray retirement as one long period of pleasure and play. Do you feel that God is calling you to a life of uninterrupted leisure or a spiritual life based on sharing your God-given gifts?

f) If you have time, watch *The Best Exotic Marigold Hotel.* Or plan to gather together again for an evening to watch and discuss this delightful film. Pay special attention to Evelyn Greenslade, the character played by Judi Dench. How does Evelyn find meaning and purpose in her new life?

Chapter 2:
Dismantling the House

So, You've Retired! Congratulations—Maybe!

You're overjoyed! Retirement at last! No wonder you are excited. This is the day you've been waiting for. You've worked hard for three, maybe four decades, or more. You've earned it. No more early mornings with the alarm ringing in your ears. No more late-night meetings. No more deadlines. No more stress related to office politics. No more worrying about performance reviews. You're free! Free to do whatever you like—to play golf or tennis at will, to spend time with the grandchildren, to enjoy winters in Florida and summers at the cottage—with even more opportunities to golf. What could be better than that?

Maybe a lot of things.

There is a wonderful film that everyone should watch more than once before they retire: *About Schmidt.*[27] With stellar performances by Jack Nicholson and Kathy Bates, as well as a good supporting cast, this movie is a must-see for those who find themselves facing retirement.

---

27   *About Schmidt,* directed by Alexander Payne (Montreal: Alliance Atlantis, 2010), DVD.

The protagonist is Warren Schmidt, a middle-management employee and actuary at Woodmen of the World, an insurance company in Omaha, Nebraska. After a brutal retirement dinner in a dingy hall on a cold, wet, dark night, accompanied by all the usual clichés and boring platitudes that often accompany such events, Schmidt goes home with his wife Helen only to face the most difficult job of his life: the transition into retirement.

Schmidt feels unappreciated and demeaned by having been replaced at his job by an inexperienced university graduate who is half his age. The humiliation is complete when he discovers his boxes of neatly packed file folders, the culmination of years of dedicated service and hard work, unceremoniously marked for the rubbish bin. His hopes of greater success and recognition now dashed, he begins to lament his only claim to fame, which was making it to a small corner of the office newsletter, the *Woodmen's Weekly Bugle* and not the much-dreamt-of cover of *Fortune* magazine.

At home, he seems to be even less appreciated. Having thrown his whole being into his work for so many years, he doesn't know what to do and feels totally useless just moping around the house. Nor does he even really know his wife of forty-two years, so defined has his life always been by the job. "Who is this old woman next to me in bed?" he asks himself. And yet when Helen dies very suddenly, his life is plunged into another abyss. Even as ineffectual as his marriage and career were, they filled a void of his life, and when both suddenly disappeared, Schmidt finds himself sinking into a deep depression.

The rest of the film describes a sad but also often hilarious journey across the country in a top-of-the-line Winnebago that Schmidt's wife had purchased—against his wishes, of course—for their retirement years. But the road trip is really a metaphor for the journey Schmidt takes to discover who he is. In the last scene of the film, one is left feeling that there is indeed hope for this pathetic, lonely man. Schmidt bursts into tears upon receiving the gift of a simple but beautiful coloured picture from his young foster child in Tanzania, in which the little boy has drawn Schmidt and himself, depicted by two smiling stick figures, one large and one small. The two are holding hands and, in contrast to the darkness and gloom of the opening scene of the film, the sun is shining brightly.

Schmidt's Question is Our Question, Too

Schmidt does not actually utter the words, but what he is thinking is self-evident. If he were to put his thoughts into words, they would sound something like this: "I don't even know who I am anymore without my job."

Recently, my husband and I ran into an old friend at the cinema. His wife said how much she was looking forward to retiring in another year or two. Then she laughed and said, "But my father (a United Church minister) is still working at eighty-seven. In fact, he helped to conduct a funeral this very morning!" I chuckled and replied, "Well, maybe that's why he is still so healthy. The work is doing him some good." Immediately, her husband interjected a much more serious tone into our conversation: "I think you are right. My fifty-seven-year-old brother retired two years ago and now he's absolutely lost."

Other people have expressed this feeling of "lostness," using words like:

> "If I'm not his wife, her husband, her wife, or his partner, who am I?"

"The loss of our house in the fire made me feel as though I'd lost a piece of myself."

"With our last child off to university, we don't feel like the same people anymore."

"Who am I now?"

"Without my job, I feel that I have lost my anchor."

In a CBC radio interview featuring journalist Jonathan Chevreau, the writer made the point that the average full-time employee works approximately 2,000 hours in a year. As he says, it's little wonder that the newly retired find themselves suffering what author Manfred F. R. Kets de Vries refers to as "retirement syndrome."[28]

Even if, unlike Schmidt, we have been blessed with a fulfilling job and a happy marriage, we can relate to his pain. Indeed, the sense of emptiness may be greater for us if only because we found these things to be so satisfying. Without the anchor of meaningful work, we, too, may find ourselves asking: Who am I?

William Bridges' Change Theory

Back in 1991, William Bridges published his now-classic *Managing Transitions*, in which he outlined a change model for businesses and organizations that were going through transition.[29] His model is very

---

28   Jonathan Chevreau in CBC interview with guest host Scott Regehr, "Victory Lap Retirement: Work While You Play, Play While You Work. The Joy of Financial Independence..."on *Metro Morning* with Matthew Galloway, January 3, 2017.

29   William Bridges, *Transitions: Making Sense of Life's Changes*, 2nd ed. (Cambridge: Da Capo Press, 2004).

helpful as we consider the way we navigate life after fifty. Bridges' change theory was born out of an experience that happened to him when he was actually much younger, about age thirty-eight or thirty-nine. He chose to give up a position he had held as an English professor at a small but reputable college in California. He and his wife, along with a group of their closest friends, decided to move to the country to live in a kind of commune. This was something he was looking forward to doing. He would enjoy growing much of the food they would eat and tending to the garden. He thought he would also have time to write, something he loved to do. So, naturally, he was very confused to discover that, when he got to the country and into his tightly knit group of friends, the first thing he experienced was a painful sense of loss. His old friends and neighbours were puzzled, too, because they knew how much he had wanted this move. Everyone was surprised by the fact that he was now just moping around acting grief-stricken instead of enjoying his newfound freedom.

One day shortly after they had arrived at their new community, Bridges' youngest daughter, Margaret, came home from the second grade to say that her teacher had asked all the students to find out what kind of work their parents did. She already knew that her mother was a counsellor, but what was Dad? Bridges said he groped for an answer, rambling on about doing some speaking and doing some writing and doing a lot of gardening and raising a few chickens. "Margaret's eyes glazed over. She was looking for a noun — *teacher, farmer, carpenter, doctor, waiter*— but the best her Dad could give her was a string of participles: doing this and doing that. Participles didn't answer her question, *What are you?*"[30]

---

30   William Bridges, *The Way of Transition* (Cambridge, Da Capo Press, 2001), 9.

SHEILA MACDONALD MACGREGOR

What he was, he realised, was a person *in transition*. And that's what many of us are, too: in transition or looking at transitions down the road.

A quick definition: According to Bridges, transition is different from change. Change is something that *happens to people*, even if they don't agree with it. They lose their job, or there is a change in management or in reporting relationships. They move to a new city. A child leaves home. A marriage ends. Transition, on the other hand, is internal: *It's what happens in people's minds and hearts as they go through these changes.*[31]

Transitions are characterized by the same three phases. Bridges describes these phases as: (1) endings, which are followed by (2) a neutral zone, the time between the old life and the new, and (3) a new beginning. All transitions, Bridges says, follow a similar cycle, taking us from endings, through emptiness and darkness, to fresh life and new beginnings. As he notes, we've all seen this pattern in nature. This movement reminds us of the cyclical nature of life: the changing seasons, the ebb and flow of the ocean tides, and the waxing and waning of the moon.

In the ending, we lose or let go of our old outlook, our old reality, our old attitudes, our old values, our old self-image. We may resist this ending for a while. We may try to talk ourselves out of what we are feeling, and when we do give in, we may be swept by feelings of sadness or anger, like Bridges himself was when he left his teaching job for a place in the country, or like Schmidt was when he retired from the job that had provided him with purpose and routine. A common question of this phase is: Why is this happening to me?[32]

---

31   Bridges, *Transitions,* 128.

32   Ibid.

What's happening, if we return to Bateson's image of the house, is that the house that we call our life is being dismantled. Not just the bricks and mortar, but the basic structure and contours of our life are suddenly being ripped away from under us. The result is that we don't know who we are anymore.

Next, we find ourselves in the neutral zone between the old and the new. This confusing state is a time when our lives feel as though they have broken apart or flat-lined. We get mixed signals, some from our old way of being and some from a way of being that is still unclear to us. It's like living amid home renovations. There is debris everywhere. Nothing feels solid. Everything is up for grabs. Yet for that very reason, it is a time when we sometimes feel that anything is possible. So, the in-between time can be a very creative time, too. It's unsettling. It's a time characterized by anxiety and, often, fear; but it is a creative time, too.

Finally, we take hold of a new identity. We have a new sense of ourselves, a new outlook, and a new sense of purpose and possibility. When we have done this, we finally feel like a new chapter in our lives has started. No matter how impossible it was to imagine a future earlier, life now feels as though it is back on track again. The house we call life is taking on structure and form, and we can finally imagine finding some pleasure living in it. In other words, we have a new beginning!

Those, in a nutshell, are Bridges' three phases of transition: Endings, the Neutral Zone, Beginnings. The lived process, however, is not as simplistic as it seems.

For example, how long should you expect to spend in each phase? Bridges admits that he himself has often struggled to discern when an ending is completed and when he has been in the neutral zone long enough. Life is not as tidy or as orderly as we would like it to be. He says that people will go through each stage at their own pace. For example, those who are comfortable with the change will likely move ahead to stage three (beginnings) more quickly, while others will linger at stage one (endings) or two (neutral zone). A new beginning can happen as a result of an external cue or an inner signal. You may chance upon an old friend in the grocery store or meet the love of your life at a party you had not planned on attending. Maybe you read about an opportunity when you are flipping through a magazine while waiting to see your doctor. It can be as random as that. When you are ready for a new change, the opportunity will find you.

But the key is to be ready. Bridges rightly points out that trying to start anew without doing the hard work of endings and neutrality is a futile exercise that will only lead to more frustration in the long term. It's like the person who jumps from relationship to relationship without stopping in between to reassess why the same patterns keep occurring. But when the hard work is done, you can enter a new phase of life with energy and vigour.

Bridges emphasizes that the actual, lived process of transition is not as linear as his writings suggest. After conversing with Canadian organizational consultant Donald Skilling, he acknowledged that it is possible to find oneself in more than one of these three phases at the same time. Think of the process as more of a curve than a straight line. The three phases of transition are not always separate stages; they frequently overlap and the boundaries blur. For example, you find yourself feeling both anxious and sad as you contemplate the end of a deeply satisfying career, while at the same time feeling genuine excitement about the possibilities this ending may bring.[33]

Bridges' Five Ds of Endings: Disengagement, Dismantling, Dis-identification, Disenchantment, & Disorientation

In this chapter, we focus on the "endings."[34] According to Bridges, endings are generally characterized in five ways: disengagement, dismantling, dis-identification, disenchantment, and disorientation.

1. Disengagement or Leaving Home

Bridges notes that it seems to be a universal belief among traditional peoples that at times of inner transition, people need to be separated from their families and communities. For example, many aboriginal tribes of Australia, and many Native North American tribes, have had a practice of sending their young men into the wilderness for up to six months to test whether they are ready to become men. Often, they are circumcised first, a tooth might be knocked out, and their faces and bodies whitened with clay so that they are no longer recognisable. The boys must survive, unassisted, and keep themselves totally isolated. When they return after several months they will be considered men of the tribe. But they are no longer the people they once were. Those young lads are now dead. Their parents signify their deaths by burning the sleeping mats they had used throughout their childhoods. When they return to the village, they will not even recognise them—at least not at first, because they are no longer theirs. In the first few weeks of

---

33   Ibid.

34   Bridges, *Transitions*.

their new life back in the village, they will not even remember their old names. They have been reborn and given a new calling.[35]

Recall the story of Jesus being tempted in the wilderness. It is such an important story that in the church we make a point of reading it every year at the beginning of Lent, when Jesus begins his journey to the cross in Jerusalem. It, too, is a story about Jesus leaving home, leaving his family and his village, wrestling with the challenges that come from living in isolation in the desert, and then emerging as a man who has been given a mission.

Disengagement or separation from the norm happens when couples separate or get divorced, when a loved one dies, when you or your partner becomes ill, when you move to a new community, when you take up a new job or leave a job, when you retire, or when the kids leave home, as well as many other events that disengage you from the contexts in which you have known yourself.

I still recall how much I sobbed and how frightened I was when I finally left home and my parents dropped me off at grad school, which, believe it or not, was the first time I had ever lived away from home. The surroundings were new, and I didn't know a soul. Without the familiarity of home and family and friends, I didn't know who I was anymore, and I was afraid. Years later, I watched helplessly as my husband and I dropped our tearful daughter off for her first year at Queen's University and, even though I knew Alexandra would make new friends in time, I was revisited by all those painful feelings I had felt nearly thirty years earlier.

---

35   Bridges, *Transitions,* 101; Bridges, *The Way of Transition,* 115.

However, I also knew that there would be other endings in her life that would hurt deeply, too. I knew this because I had been there on more than one occasion. I felt it when the young man I dated all through high school and university and I parted company. I felt genuine sorrow when I left behind my seminary years at Princeton, with all their intellectual stimulation and the wonderful friends I had made there, and embarked on my first real job. I felt it whenever I left behind a congregation I loved and served to take up ministry with a new congregation I did not yet know. I experienced it much more deeply when my parents died, my aunts passed away, and when I lost a much-beloved friend to cancer.

Children can experience this, too. I remember the first time I felt so bereft occurred when I was only thirteen. My best friend Elizabeth was moving away, and I just could not imagine never walking home from school with her again and chatting about all the things young girls on the cusp of adolescence talk about. I could not imagine entering that huge secondary school the following autumn without a familiar face by my side. I missed my old school, my friends, and my teachers. In fact, I came home every day of my first year of high school and wept buckets. I was devastated. I didn't stop crying until Christmas, which is when I met my new friends Carla, Helga, and the two Judys.

2. Dismantling

Remember our metaphor about renovating our house? Endings involve a dismantling of the house we call our life. Like the house under renovation, this is when our lives become completely dismantled; when we're stripped right down to the studs and the boards. This is the grieving process.

This is where we find Schmidt. He is in grief, mourning the loss of his old life where everything was known and familiar. Now his life has been stripped right down to the studs. And as the contractors always warn you, remodeling always takes more time and money than new construction. This is good advice for anyone in transition, too. That's why Bridges says the common mistake of people entering retirement is that they rush into being busy. Don't rush this ending period. Likewise, people often make the mistake of rushing into a new marriage after their partner has died. While this is true of both men and women, it can be especially true of men. My mother and my aunts used to have a saying: "Women grieve; men remarry." But male, female or transgendered, if you don't do the important work of grieving first, you may put your second relationship in jeopardy. As the author of the 23rd Psalm writes, you must go "through the valley of the shadow of death" in order to arrive at the other side. You can't go around it or above it or below it. You have to go *through* it. There is no way to avoid the valley and the hard work that endings demand. Sadly, this is a biblical truth that we in the advantaged part of the world love to deny, at our own peril.

3. Dis-identification

When you become separated from your old community, whether it be a physical place or a marriage, you also lose your old ways of identifying yourself. Many experience this as a loss of role that prescribed their behaviour and made them feel identifiable. No longer being Bob's wife, Jim's husband, or Amanda's mother; no longer a teacher or lawyer or nurse or construction worker or the vice-president of marketing. Feeling that you no longer have an identity. Again, that question that troubled Schmidt: Who am I, now that I am no longer defined by the job or the kids or by what I did? Interestingly, this is the theme of many films today directed at those in the second half of life. Recall the poignant lament of the once-popular opera diva Jean Horton, played by actor Maggie Smith in *Quartet*: "You need to understand that I was someone once!"[36]

Christensen says that the fact that most retired people continue to identify themselves by the job they *used to do*—I am a retired dentist, a retired banker, a retired electrician, a retired hairdresser—suggests that they have not done the hard work of looking deeply into themselves to learn who they are and where they are being called in this new phase of life.[37] And no doubt about it: "identity work" is hard slogging! Scott Peck, the author of the acclaimed book, *The Road Less Traveled*, once observed that most Westerners are just spiritually lazy and thus are not prepared to do the difficult and often time-consuming work necessary to discern who they really are.[38] Yet, again and again, we see how essential it is to devote some serious time to this task. Moreover, this is holy work. In the scriptures, it is only after many hours of nocturnal wrestling in the wilderness with the angel that Jacob is given a new identity and becomes Israel (Genesis 32:26–32).

If you want to know who you are, you need to do the hard work of introspection.

4. Disenchantment

If the first half of life, especially our first twenty years, is about learning new things, the second half is often about *unlearning* things. This is when

---

36   *Quartet*, directed by Dustin Hoffman (Headline Pictures, BBC Films, DCM Productions, 2012), film.

37   Janet Christensen interview.

38   M. Scott Peck, *The Road Less Travelled.* (New York, Touchstone Books, 1978), pp. 269-270.

you realise that some significant part of your old reality was in your head, not out there. The flawless parent, the noble leader, the perfect spouse, the wonderful boss, and the utterly trustworthy friend. It's also, I suspect, a time when we must come to grips with our disappointment with our own selves. Later in the movie, for example, Schmidt comes to a place where he is able to admit to himself: "Maybe I wasn't the greatest husband. Maybe I could have treated Helen better."[39]

Most of us have experienced disappointments in life. Like Schmidt, many of us harbour some regrets about the way we have lived or treated others. The crowd that watched Jesus's crucifixion knew this kind of sorrow and remorse on a very deep level. Luke writes: "When all the people who had gathered to witness this sight saw what took place, they went home beating their breasts" (Luke 23:48). In other words, they went away feeling guilty. Would that they would have heard Jesus's words from the cross: "Father, forgive them, for they know not what they do" (Luke 23:34)? Guilt is paralyzing; forgiveness is empowering. Coming to a place where we can accept Christ's forgiveness and learn to forgive ourselves is part of the important work we must learn to do when we are in transition, especially when we find ourselves in the place of disenchantment.

Sometimes disenchantment is more about coming to the recognition that the things to which you devoted the bulk of your time and energy in the first half of life are not, to a large degree, things that have any lasting significance.[40] In the scramble to build a career or create a home, it's possible to lose sight of those things that really and truly and ultimately matter. The

39   *About Schmidt.* DVD. Directed by Alexander Payne. Alliance Atlantis, Montreal, 2010.

40   Dr. Anne Beattie-Stokes, in Correspondence to author, April 2017.

extra space provided by the atrium of life can give you the room and the time you need to reflect more deeply on the choices you have made and how you want to live your life going forward.

The good news about disenchantment, Bridges says, whether suffering from a minor disappointment or a major shock, is that it is often a signal that things are moving into transition. That something is ending, and that maybe it is time to look beneath the surface of our lives. Perhaps this is why Stevens refers to retirement "as a useful shock."[41] It forces people to look beneath the surface of their lives and really consider where and how God is calling them to serve.

5. *Disorientation*

Bridges describes the final stage of endings in this way:

> The "reality" that is left behind in all endings is not just a picture on the wall. It is a sense of which way is up and which way is down. It is a sense of which way is forward and which way is back. It is, in short, a way of orienting oneself and of moving forward into the future. In the old passage or initiation rituals, the one in transition would often be taken into unfamiliar territory, beyond the bounds of former experience, and left there for a time. All customary signs of location would be gone and the only remaining source of orientation would be the heavens. This is the part of the ending process where we feel most lost, confused, and where we have that don't-know-where-I-am feeling. The old

---

41   R. Paul Stevens, *Work Matters,* Loc. 120 of 1854.

sense that life as "going somewhere" breaks down, and we feel like shipwrecked sailors on some existential island. Things that used to be important don't seem to matter much now. We feel stuck, dead, lost in some great, dark world.[42]

Like Schmidt, we feel like we are living through our own funeral. Like Jesus being tempted by the devil in the desert, we often feel overwhelmed, lost in a spiritual wasteland. Like the people of Israel roaming around the wilderness, with the familiarly of Pharaoh's Egypt behind them and the promise of the Land of Milk and Honey still far off in the distance, we feel like the future isn't anywhere. *We don't know who we are. The house that is our life is crumbling down round about us. Life, as we know it, is ending.*

In the End is Our Beginning

"Now among those who went up to worship at the festival were some Greeks. [21] They came to Philip, who was from Bethsaida in Galilee, and said to him, "Sir, we wish to see Jesus." [22] Philip went and told Andrew; then Andrew and Philip went and told Jesus. [23] Jesus answered them, "The hour has come for the Son of Man to be glorified. [24] Very truly, I tell you, unless a grain of wheat falls into the earth and dies, it remains just a single grain; but if it dies, it bears much fruit. [25] Those who love their life lose it, and those who hate their life in this world will keep it for eternal life. [26] Whoever serves me must follow me, and where I am, there will

---

42   Bridges, *Transitions,* 101.

my servant be also. Whoever serves me, the Father
will honor."

– John 12:20–26

The bible talks a lot about endings. More importantly, it reminds us
that endings are essential if something new is going to be born in our
life. In the above passage, Jesus says: "Very truly, I tell you, unless a
grain of wheat falls into the earth and dies, it remains just a single
grain; but if it dies, it bears much fruit."

Saint Paul gives emphasis to Jesus's teaching. In his Letter to the
Romans, he writes: "Therefore we have been buried with him by
baptism into death, so that, just as Christ was raised the dead by the
glory of the Father, so we too might walk in newness of life." (Romans
6:4). Again, to the Corinthians, Paul writes: "What you sow does not
come to life unless it dies" (I Corinthians 15:36).

The New Testament is very clear. Dying to self (self-centredness) is
never portrayed in scripture as something optional in the Christian
life. Sometimes a relationship needs to die for something new and
better to be born. In my twenties, I had to leave behind a relationship
that had become comfortable yet sterile to pursue a calling that has
brought my life enormous satisfaction and meaning, not to mention
a life partner who has brought me more joy than I could ever have
imagined. As well, sometimes, we must lose old habits and old ways
of being in order to be born again. For something new to be born,

something needs to die first. As Natalie Sleeth wrote in her beautiful hymn: "In our end is our beginning."[43]

There's a wonderful film that underscores this truth. Premiering in 1988 and starring Dustin Hoffman and Tom Cruise, the film is called *Rain Man*.[44] The story centres around baby boomer Charlie Babbitt (played by Cruise), who is a selfish, hustling salesman. Hoffman plays his older autistic brother, Raymond who had been institutionalized. Ironically, Charlie didn't even know he had an older brother, much less an autistic one, and the only reason he acknowledges him now is that their father has died and left $3 million to autistic Raymond and an old '49 Buick to hotshot Charlie. Charlie spends most of his time moving in on poor Raymond to manipulate and cheat him out of the inheritance. He can't imagine that Raymond would know what to do with all that money, but Charlie can sure think of a few things. So, he goes after Raymond to get the money. But during the movie, against his will, Charlie begins to develop a fondness—a deep fondness—for his older brother. And before he knows it, for the first time in his life, Charlie is thinking more of another human being than of himself. Slowly, he begins to die to self and live for Raymond. Thus, he changes. He becomes a different person, a whole new human being[45]. But he had to die to his old self to be redeemed and reborn. As the old Charlie dies, a new Charlie is born. In his end, he discovers a new beginning and a reason to live. His transformation calls to mind Jesus's

---

43   Natalie Sleeth, *In the Bulb There is A Flower.* (Carol Stream, Illinois, Hope Publishing Company, 1986.)

44   *Rain Man*, directed by Barry Levinson (1988).

45   William J. Bausch, *More Telling Stories. More Compelling Stories.* (Mystic, Connecticut, Twenty-Third Publication, 1993), p. 97.

words: "Those who love their life will lose it, and those who hate their life in this world will keep it for eternal life." (John 12:25)

Right now, we are people in transition, struggling with the endings of life, be that the end of a career we loved, an empty nest, or the end of a relationship that brought our lives meaning and purpose. As the house we call our life seems to be dismantling around about us, we need to consider what we are willing to lose in order that something new might be built. The questions we must ask ourselves at each of life's endings are: What must we let go of to grow? For whose sake will we give our lives in order that we might be born anew? These are questions we will wrestle with in the next chapters.

For Further Reading:

William Bridges, *Transitions: Making Sense of Life's Changes*, 2nd Edition. (Cambridge, DaCapo Press, 2004.)

For Viewing:

About Schmidt, Director Alexander Payne, 2002.

Re-Designing Your Life: A Practical Spirituality for the Second Half of Life. Sheila Macdonald Macgregor, Wib Dawson, videographer and editor, 2017.

Questions for Discussion:

Watch Session Two of the videos that have been made to accompany this book and then discuss the following. Note: if you are leading a study group, you may not have time to discuss all the questions. Choose those that you feel will be most helpful to your group.

1. Describe a time in your life when something you valued came to an end. Consider using a pencil, coloured markers, watercolour crayons, or clay to express how you felt. Or try writing a poem or setting your thoughts to music or dance. Share with the group as you are comfortable.

2. How did you cope, or not cope, at the time? Where did you draw strength from to help you deal with the pain you experienced? (You may wish to use a similar creative approach to respond to these questions.)

3. Read Matthew 3:13–4:11. When Jesus left home, he was baptized by John the Baptist in the Jordan River and then sent out into the wilderness for a period of testing.

a) What lessons did Jesus learn in the desert and how can these help us as we enter the second half of life?

b) Though we, too, must wrestle in our own wildernesses, what comfort can we draw from Matthew 4:11? Who are the angels who have come to you in your times of ending?

3. Read Psalm 23. Think of a time when you failed to grieve an ending in your life and instead tried to bypass a "valley." Why is it important for us to "go through the valley" and not around it? Who promises to be with us when we travel through the dark and frightening valleys of life?

d) Instead of seeing ourselves as being a "retired (you fill in the blank)," what happens when we begin to see ourselves the way Christ sees us, as his beloved friends? "I no longer call you servants, because a servant does not know his master's business. Instead, I have called you friends, for everything that I learned from my Father I have made known to you" (John 15:15, NIV).

e) Read Romans 6:4 and John 12:20-26. The bible affirms that, for something to be born, something first must die. What things in your life must you let die so that there may be rebirth?

f) If you have time, watch the film *About Schmidt*, or plan to gather together again for an evening to watch and discuss it. What things did Schmidt need to grieve or let go of to make a fresh start in life? What things do you need to grieve or let go of and how will you find forgiveness so that you can move forward into the life that God wants to give you?

Chapter 3:
Living in Chaos—
Surviving Home Renovations

Welcome to the Neutral Zone!

When I was a teenager, one of my mother's dearest friends died. Gwyn was a beautiful woman, both inside and out. She was also a beautiful seamstress and talented artistically, and hence a great loss both to her church and community. But her untimely death at the age of fifty-three was an even greater blow to her friends and family. Her husband, Joe, to whom she had been married for nearly thirty years, was especially devastated. Both of their children were in their mid-twenties and had left home a few years before. He and Gwyn were just beginning to enjoy the fruits of their hard-earned labours, and then she suddenly became very ill and died. Without his loving partner by his side, Joe no longer knew who he was. His house had just come tumbling down, and he couldn't put the pieces back together again. So, he did the only thing he could think to do. To ease his loneliness and fear, he began dating and, in no time, he was married again. About six months after his marriage to another lovely woman, my mother ran into Joe downtown one afternoon. He looked lost and forlorn. The reason was simple, as he discovered too late. His new wife was a fine woman, but she wasn't Gwyn.

Nowadays, Joe would have been encouraged to seek grief counselling; but forty years ago, such therapeutic interventions were still in their infancy and not widely available. Raised in a time when men were supposed to be strong and independent, who knows whether Joe would have even availed himself of such services? If he had, he might have learned that endings take time because grief takes time.

This is true whether we are talking about the end of an important relationship through death or divorce, or the end of a career. Authors Jack Hansen and Jerry Haas have spent years interviewing retired men and women and one of the things they have noticed is the tendency of newly retired people to "throw [themselves] into busy work to avoid the feelings of loss, emptiness, and lack of direction."[46] Canadian retirement coach Janet Christensen calls this "retirement by default."[47] For this reason, Marc Freedman, a leading expert on the longevity revolution and the transformation of retirement, argues that what most retirees need is a "grown-up gap year,"[48] where they undertake no major commitments and join no major committees for one whole year. This way, they have the time they need to really discern their callings. While it may not be a practical solution for everyone, there are ways to undertake a modified version of Freedman's "gap year." Hansen and Haas, for example, strongly recommend doing nothing for at least the first few months after retirement and, instead, just living with the feelings of loss that may surface during this period.[49] Keeping a journal during this

---

46   R. Jack Hansen and Jerry P Haas, *Retirement as Spiritual Pilgrimage: Stories, Scripture & Practices for the Journey.* (CreateSpace Independent Publishing, 2015), e-book, Location 446.

47   Janet Christensen Interview.

48   Glenn Hodges, "Interview with Marc Freedman on the Midlife Crisis: 'The Big Shift' argues for a new life stage," *AARP Bulletin*, May 12, 2011.

49   R. Jack Hansen and Jerry P Haas, *Retirement as Spiritual Pilgrimage*, Location 464.

often emotionally difficult but necessary time, they believe, can be a very helpful tool as people contemplate where and how God is calling them into the future. Their advice echoes that of Bridges, who urges people to live with the endings, not to rush them. This is what the Neutral Zone is all about.

Don't Rush Through the Neutral Zone

Bridges notes that the Neutral Zone is the time when the real business of transition takes place. While it represents probably the toughest journey any of us will ever take, the reality is that this is where the true work of transformation happens. Looking back, people often say that "everything happened back then—even though, at the time, I didn't know what was going on."[50] Again, it is important that we take time to really live in the Neutral Zone and not rush things. Too often, in our society, we want the quick fix. But as the saying goes, "No pain, no gain."

This often tends to be a very lonely time for many people. Most relationships forged in the workplace tend to fade after retirement and need to be replaced. So often people feel lost and lonesome during this period. Remember the passage journey we talked about in the previous chapter? The old passage rituals provided the young person with an experience of deep aloneness by sending him out into the wilderness. Interestingly, the Hebrew word for the "wilderness" in which Jesus, Moses, and Buddha spent time during critical periods of their lives is the same word that means "sanctuary." Do you remember what God said to Moses at the burning bush?

---

50   Bridges, *Transitions,* 154.

> When the Lord saw that he had turned aside to see, God called to him out of the bush, "Moses, Moses!" And he said, "Here I am." [5] Then he said, "Come no closer! Remove the sandals from your feet, for the place on which you are standing is holy ground." [6] He said further, "I am the God of your father, the God of Abraham, the God of Isaiah, and the God of Jacob." And Moses hid his face, for he was afraid to look at God.
>
> (Exodus 3:4–6).

It was in the wilderness that Moses found Holy Ground and, ultimately, God. Later, in chapter 20, we learn just how bleak a place this was for Moses, not only in terms of the barren geography but also emotionally and spiritually: "...Moses drew near unto the thick darkness where God was" (Exodus 20:21). Think of it. What a place to find God! And yet, again and again, this is exactly where people have experienced the divine and found themselves spiritually nourished and enriched. United Church minister Anne Beattie-Stokes underwent a huge transformation in her faith and spirituality during a retreat on Antelope Island in the Great Salt Lake. Happening upon the beauty and stillness of a dead doe in a stand of pampas grass, Anne came to see that God was calling her to a new a ministry: "to help create a safe place for people to die."[51]

The historian Arnold Toynbee pointed out that most great creative individuals in history have withdrawn to some lonely place on the eve

---

51   Anne Beattie-Stokes, *A Heart of Wisdom: Inspiration and Instruction for Conscious Elderhood.* (North Charleston, SC: Booksurge Publishing, 2009), 7, 20–21, 23.

of their rebirth. He called this "the pattern of withdrawal and return," and he traced it out in the lives of Jesus, St. Paul, St. Benedict, Gregory the Great, the Buddha, Muhammad, Dante, and others.[52]

The Neutral Zone is the time between the old life and the new. As such, it is or can be a particularly rich time for developing new insights about our lives. It's a time of inner reorientation, a kind of fallow time in our lives. Think of it as a time-out. To use the metaphor of the house again, while it is heartbreaking to find the home that was our life in ruins, there is now the opportunity not only to rebuild, but also to be our own architect and fashion a life that is uniquely ours. As Christensen teaches, this is "retirement by design, not default!"[53]

Find Meaning in Your Smaller World

In working with clients struggling to make sense of their lives in retirement, Christensen identifies several key changes that occur in people's lives when they leave their jobs. Not only is there a loss of income, which many people anticipate and plan for, but there are also things that they don't anticipate. There is the loss of meaningful activity that gives their lives both structure and purpose.

In June of 2015, Fran Boone retired from a very fulfilling career of forty-two years as a registered nurse. As she recounts, her decision was not an easy one. "My nursing career," she writes, "provided me with a great deal of satisfaction from taking care of patients."[54] Most

52   Arnold Toynbee, *A Study of History: Abridgement of Volumes 1-6* (Oxford: Oxford University Press, 1947), 577; Bridges, *Transitions*, 155.

53   Janet Christensen interview.

54   Fran Boone, Interview on December 12, 2016, London, Ontario, and email to author from Fran Boone, December 13, 2016.

of her career was spent in the highly demanding field of hemodialysis. When she began her career in dialysis back in 1978 at University Hospital in London, Ont., she was the only applicant for the job. "Dialysis units were known to be high-tech and high-stress areas to work." Fran enjoyed the challenge and especially found meaning in helping the patients. As time passed, however, she found herself more fatigued and less able to cope with the pressures. She realised that it was time to retire. What she had not counted on was the emptiness she would experience following the initial honeymoon phase of retirement. Without a regular structure to her day, Fran found herself in a deep spiritual depression only six months after she left her position at University Hospital. While her body was telling her that it was time to step back from full-time work, the decision to retire had left her without a reason to get up in the morning. She was in crisis.

In addition to the loss of a regular routine, retirement can also bring the loss of status. Along with this, there is the loss of recognition and appreciation that often go with one's work and position. As Fran also discovered, the world shrinks in one other important way that people don't often consider when they prepare to retire: the loss of contact with workmates and colleagues.[55]

This is important. Indeed, more significant than even the change of routine, is connection to other people. Many former relationships end, or at least change. I remember a former director of a board of education, a highly respected man in our community, telling me that his greatest surprise about retirement was that relationships changed.

---

55   Janet Christensen Interview.

Friendships at work that he had expected to maintain in retirement came to an end, while other relationships grew or developed.[56]

This is also true of our personal or family relationships. One person's transition can put everyone within a family into transition, too. Often this can result in good changes. For example, many people report developing closer relationships with siblings after they retire or become empty nesters.

But retirement can also impact relationships in challenging ways. Whenever a member of a system changes, the other members will feel a twinge. Children are bothered when divorced or widowed parents begin to date again. Siblings conspire to keep one another in line long after they have stopped living under the same roof. And, of course, partners in an intimate relationship react with alarm to unexpected changes in the other person.

Relationships are always structured by unspoken agreements, although people are seldom conscious of it. Beginning very early there is a psychological division of labour within a relationship. One person takes care of the financial issues, and the other handles the relationship issues; or one expresses emotions and the other anchors the relationship in practical ways. In my own household, it is generally understood that I will look after making all the doctors' appointments, booking theatre tickets, inviting friends or family for dinner, and arranging holidays and trips. I will take care of those matters that involve phone arrangements or emails. I will also look after sending cards and purchasing gifts for birthdays, christenings, weddings, anniversaries, and Christmas. Richard looks after the

---

56 Conversation with Jack Little, former Director of the London Board of Education, September 2014.

yard work, gets the kids to their hockey games and other activities, and does most of the cooking and a fair bit of the laundry, since I am often at evening meetings. He likes to cook, and he has more time than me to take care of the laundry! It will be interesting to see, though, what happens when I retire, which I will do five years before Richard.

It is not uncommon for roles to change when one or more partners retire. When my mother-in-law retired two years before my father-in-law, she was not well pleased when he left her with all the household chores instead of continuing to share in them as he had done before she retired. On the other hand, by the time he retired two years later, he was surprised—and not a little disconcerted—to discover that his wife had built a whole life for herself outside the home and would not always be around during the day to visit with him.

When one partner is in transition, it is natural that the other partner may experience panic. It's like the anxiety an actor would feel if his cue produced no entrance and no response. Recently, I attended my youngest son's Grade 12 drama class production. Malcolm had spent hours rehearsing his lines, but the young person playing opposite him momentarily lost her place, and this threw them both off. Thankfully, the prompter fed them their lines and the play was back on track, but while there are lots of good marriage counsellors that can help couples navigate these new situations, there is no prompter on the sidelines of a marriage to help them to know how to respond to their new situation on a day-to-day basis. This is something that must be negotiated and which they must learn over time.

Paul Stevens says that we must be prepared to get married again and again as we age. He does not mean we should chuck the spouse of our youth—far from it! What he means is that we must continually renegotiate our marriage as we grow older. He says: "My wife is not the woman I married over fifty years ago, and I am certainly not the man she married."[57]

Sometimes, the second one to retire unconsciously places expectations on their partner to be available to him or her to do things and go places that were not possible when working full time. For example, a woman retired two years before her husband. By the time he retired, his wife had already developed her own routine. I remember she said to me: "When my husband retired it was just like having a big black spider sitting in the corner watching me all the time!" Now she sends him off on errands every day and since he is fortunate to run into people he knows all over their small town, he is often gone for hours—and out of her hair for hours, too!

When I was young, my parents used to make a point of hiring a baby-sitter, usually my cousin, to come and watch my brother and me while they went out on a date. Mom called this "marriage insurance." When I married, she reminded me that this kind of insurance was essential to a healthy marriage, and I agree. Many times in our married life, my husband, Richard, and I have not been able to afford anything more than a coffee and a muffin at Tim Horton's, but it's not the price of the meal that matters. It's the time that's spent together. As couples retire, they may find that they need to draw on this insurance to a greater degree. For example, some couples agree to dedicate two days a week just for themselves. You may choose to call this "date time." Others

---

57   R. Paul Stevens, Interview, October 25th, 2016, Regent College Vancouver, British Columbia.

may agree to schedule individual activities Monday through Thursday, keeping Friday through Sunday as their time together. I know of one couple that agreed that they would not expect to eat breakfast or lunch together, but that suppers would always be shared with each other. As one woman said, "I married him for love, not for lunch!"[58]

All kidding aside, marriage *post-kids and post-career* can be hard work for many couples. Two years ago, a woman in my congregation came to me, very concerned about her cousin and his wife. They had been married for over thirty years, their kids were grown and on their own, and now, after three-and-a-half decades in the workforce, they decided to retire and together build the home of their dreams on the small northern lake where they had enjoyed many pleasant summer vacations. They spent two years building their dream house, and it was beautiful. Once they had moved and got settled in their new home, they found themselves in marriage counselling, wondering if there was any future for their marriage or not.

According to Wendy Dennis in a recent article posted by Zoomer Media, their situation is not unusual. "In Canada, divorce is spiking only among fifty-plusers and becoming an increasingly common event for couples sixty-five and older. . .. The trend is so striking it has been dubbed the 'grey divorce revolution.'"[59] Dennis also notes that this phenomenon is not limited to the Western world. Even in traditional Japan, there has been an increase in the divorce rate among older adults. The latter is often attributed to "retired husband syndrome,"

---

58   Or "I married him for better or worse – but not for lunch." Hazel Weiss, in Mary Catherine Bateson *Composing a Further Life*, 19.

59   Wendy Dennis, *"How Grey Divorce Became the New Normal,"* June 3, 2016, Posted by Zoomer Media Limited, 2017.

where Japanese wives have been shown to suffer from both physical illness and depression because of the constant nagging of their newly retired bored and grumpy husbands.[60] This may be cause for alarm, but it is not a reason to throw in the towel. According to Christensen, if couples are prepared to do the hard inner work that retirement (and marriage in retirement) requires, they may be able to build an even deeper and stronger marital relationship.

Whatever challenges couples face in the second half of life, there is no question that for many of them, post-retirement marriage represents "an ongoing adjustment and work in progress."[61] Marriage relationships in the early stages of retirement can sometimes be strained not only by the absence of outside schedules, but also by the reality that both are trying to figure out "who we are in this new stage of life." What Bateson says about aging, in general, is especially true of marriage in the retirement years: It "has become an improvisational art form calling for imagination and willingness to learn. . .. To know what they will need and what they need to offer, both men and women must explore who they are."[62] The key—as in many other aspects of life (married or otherwise)—is communication. Talk about your expectations and feelings. And do this *before* you retire!

---

60   Marco Bertoni and Giorgio Brunell, "Pappa Ante Portas: The Retired Husband Syndrome in Japan," DISCUSSION PAPER SERIES, Forschungsinstitut zur Zukunft der Arbeit, Institute for the Study of Labor, IZA DP No. 8350 July 2014.

61   Interview with Karen and Bill Butt, October 21, 2016, London, Ont.

62   Bateson, *Composing a Further Life. The Age of Active Wisdom*, p. 19.

Keep Connecting to Your Changing Relationships

There are also, of course, many blessings that come to women and men in retirement. There is the gift of being able to spend more time with adult children or nieces and nephews, especially if your children live a long way away and you need time to be able to travel to see them. Some couples or individuals decide to sell up and move across the country to be near their children. But this can be both a plus and a minus, especially if it means leaving behind close friends, church, and other organizations that have brought your life meaning, or if it means that you are not able to respond to God's call on your life. Karen and Bill Butt, who served as overseas personnel with the United Church of Canada in Mozambique, were taken aback by the number of friends and acquaintances who expressed disdain at their decision to accept a call to serve in southeast Africa. These people felt that Karen and Bill were shirking their responsibilities to their adult children and elderly parents. Interestingly, neither their children nor their parents felt abandoned. In fact, they took great pride in the important ministry that Karen and Bill had undertaken. Bill says the family grew stronger because they had to find more creative ways of staying in touch, like email and Skype. Moreover, their children and grandparents grew closer as they cared for one another. In serving the people of Mozambique, Karen and Bill taught their children a valuable lesson: that God's family is much bigger than our own immediate circle of blood relatives. As Jesus said: "My mother and my brothers are those who hear the word of God and do it." (Luke 8:21). Today, Bill and Karen, who are back in Canada, enjoy their visits with their grandchildren and have many rich and wonderful stories to share with them.

It's often said that "grandchildren are the reward for not having killed your kids." I have even heard it said that, if Abraham had been asked to sacrifice his grandchild instead of his son, there is no way on earth he would have done so. You might be tempted to kill your kids, but never your grandchildren!

If you missed a lot of time with your own children when they were growing up because you were busy working, you may look upon this as a very special time and an opportunity that you don't want to miss this time around. My friend Catherine frequently travels to Toronto or Ottawa to help care for her grandchildren. Pauline, whose youngest grandchild lives in the same city, dedicates two days a week to her care. Both regard these times with their little ones as a blessing of these years. Will Randolph, Director of Aging and Older Adult Ministries in the United Methodist Church and one of the founders of Boomerstock[63], sees grandparents as being key to the transmission of Christian faith and values today.[64] As he notes, grandparents who spend time with their grandchildren have a unique opportunity to share their faith with the younger generations and thus become important channels for passing on Christian beliefs and principles.

However, we all know of grandparents who never seem to have a life because their kids are always dropping the grandchildren off at their place. There are many grandparents, too, who are raising their grandchildren. In the last decade-and-a-half of my ministry, I have noticed

---

63   Boomerstock was a first-of-its kind event on Baby Boomers and Spirituality and one of the most exciting ministry initiatives to emerge out of the United Methodist Church in the USA. Its focus was to help both professionals and laypeople in the Church reach out to the Boomer generation, and to assist in building disciples among the Boomer population so that they in turn could connect with younger generations.

64   Rev. Dr. William B. Randolph, in the opening address at Boomerstock, September 26, 2016, Nashville, Tenn.

not only a sharp increase in the number of grandparents who provide full- or half-time daycare for their grandchildren, but also a major increase in the number of grandparents who are serving as surrogate parents, sometimes on their own, sometimes with one or both children's parents living in the home, creating a whole new set of dynamics and often unimaginable stress and tension for all three generations. I even had one understandably distressed grandmother tell me that her adult daughter would now be living with her every other week. Apparently, the judge presiding over her daughter's divorce case had given the parents joint custody of the children, with the caveat that the children must continue to be raised in the family home. Mom and Dad both wound up returning to their parents' homes to live during the weeks the other parent had custody!

For grandparents who find themselves in one of these situations, there is far less time to pursue the hobbies and interests in which they may have hoped to engage after retirement, especially if they have taken on childcare duties. They may even need to keep on working so that they can afford to help their adult children and grandchildren who have moved in with them. One couple, whose daughter and grandson live with them permanently, tells me that they no longer plan anything more than day trips, and even then, they fit their plans around school and after-school sports and activities. Because their daughter and grandchild both suffer from depression, they make sure that they are never more than an hour's drive from home.

Individuals and couples without children and grandchildren enter retirement with a somewhat different experience. They may feel left out as they hear their friends happily recounting the endlessly cute things their kids or grandkids get up to. On the other hand, there is much truth in what my Aunt Grace used to say, "If you don't have them (children) to make you laugh, you won't have them to make you cry."

That said, those who do not have children (or whose relations with their children are strained) may also worry about who will care for them when they need it. Craig Kennet Miller writes that the growing number of single people over the age of sixty-five can no longer count on the support of family to come to their aid when they become ill.[65] Relating to children and grandchildren may also be more complicated when they are stepchildren and step-grandchildren. And, let's face it, even when they are our own kids, this does not mean that they are going to be easy to get along with or even supportive. They may live thousands of miles away. They may be too busy to get home very often. Or they may be very demanding. A colleague of mine recently wrote to me, saying: "Don't waste a minute of your [retirement] trying to please anyone other than yourself—particularly not your children!"

Sometimes, if we are honest, our kids are not only demanding, but they are also not very nice. Indeed, our children are not all good just because they are our children. There is a tendency for us to sentimentalize our relationships with our children and grandchildren, in much the same way that one may sentimentalize one's relationship to a deceased parent or spouse. After the death of my uncle, who was a genuinely nice guy, my grieving aunt idealized her relationship with him so much that the rest of the family became convinced that Uncle Ted had now superseded Jesus at the right hand of God!

---

65   Craig Kennet Miller, *Boomer Spirituality. Seven Values for the Second Half of Life*. (Nashville, Discipleship Resources, 2016), p. 44.

Because the gift of another twenty or thirty years also means that there are more great-grandparents around, this points to another blessing of these years that can also be a challenge. Many women and men entering the second half of life are not only helping to support adult children and raise grandchildren, but they may also be caring for their own elderly parents. Little wonder that this generation has been identified as the "sandwich generation," or, as one wit has put it, "the club sandwich generation."[66]

It is no wonder that those entering the second half of life suffer from greater stress than previous generations. Between caring for elderly parents, raising children, and looking after their own demanding jobs, they face a tough balancing act. According to Dr. Richard Earle, managing director of the Canadian Institute of Stress, baby boomers have a higher rate of depression than the previous generation. As he says, "What we're noticing at the Canadian Institute of Stress and throughout the research literature is a significant rise in mood disorders, including depression, in that baby-boomer age group...."[67] Earle goes so far as to say that "it's not just a sandwich generation—it's a triple-decker sandwich because they're [boomers] looking after a husband or wife and job and the rest of it."[68]

As I look around my congregation at the women and men who are in midlife, or watch my friends cope with the needs of elderly parents, I can't help but notice the impact this has on their own quality of life.

---

66 Sandwich generation refers to those who are sandwiched in between caring for elderly parents and young children at the same time. A club sandwich happens when we find ourselves sandwiched between their own aging parents (or partners), their adult children, and their grandchildren.

67 Cindy Chan, *"Stress of Caregiving."* (Ottawa, The Epoch Times, June 8, 2010.)

68 Ibid.

Some need to take time off from work to care for their parents or even retire early. Since the majority of those who provide the caregiving are women, this often means a significant loss in income or a cut in retirement benefits. Moreover, as Christensen points out, because many of these women also took time out for maternity leaves or to raise their children, these are cuts that they can ill afford.[69] Not only this, but according to Earle, about thirty-two percent of these adult children, both men and women, say they've had to cancel travel plans, thirty-four percent have dropped personal hobbies and interests, and well over seventy percent say the balancing act is interfering with their ability to fulfill responsibilities at work. Worst of all, Earle says, many of these same people report "a feeling of not being able to find pleasure from things they used to enjoy, and within that, not being able to concentrate, to focus on what they're doing, making decisions, and certainly sleep disturbance."[70]

Worries are compounded when one cannot easily get to the parent who is ailing, especially when that parent lives in a nursing home many kilometres away and is suffering both physical and emotional pain. A sense of helplessness fuels feelings of guilt and deep sorrow, as in the case of Liz, who was limited much of the time to phone conversations or occasional weekend visits with her elderly mother, who suffered from severe depression in her final years. Before her mother died, Liz said: "I find it incredibly hard to be with her or even talk to her on the phone, as I do not have the skills to help a person with mental illness."

---

69   Christensen, interview.

70   Cindy Chan, Ibid. See also Norman De Bono, "Canadians 65 and older have highest suicide rate of any group in the country," *The London Free Press*, June 16, 2013.

Under such circumstances, it is important that we create or seek out friends and communities where we can feel supported. The latter provide some temporary structures to hold our house together when it is under renovation. Such friends and communities can also be places where we can find strength and encouragement for our own journey. Above all, they remind us that we are not alone in our journey and that others can help.

Realise the Importance of Community

When your house is in ruins, you need to be able to access good temporary shelter. As Bridges notes, when you are in transition and the house that is your life is undergoing renovation (or has just been pulled out from under you), then you need to put some temporary structures in place.

Here, it is imperative to emphasize the importance of community as we move into the second half of life. Clayton even goes so far as to say that "our choice of communities is a matter of life and death."[71] Given that isolation and loneliness have been identified as chief factors contributing to poor mental health among older adults, the findings of the Canadian Mental Health Association are alarming. In a 2012 report, the CMHA noted that those aged sixty-five and older, especially men, have a higher suicide rate than other generations. The report said that this is especially true of baby boomers.[72]

Paul Links, chief of psychiatry at the Schulich School of Medicine at Western University, says that his own extensive research in the field

---

71   Clayton, *Called for Life*, p. 47.

72   Norman De Bono, Ibid.

also bears this out.[73] He has seen the increase in depression among seniors firsthand in his practice. As he notes, men over sixty-five who have enjoyed highly successful careers are most susceptible to depression and suicide. Links points to the lack of "connectiveness," isolation, and loneliness as chief causes of deteriorating mental health among older adults. Studies also show that the rate of depression in both men and women over the age of sixty-five is twenty-five percent of the total population, which is approximately ten percent higher than the rate of depression in the population under sixty-five. We can only begin to imagine the pressure this will place on our health-care system as boomers continue to age. However, the good news is that we can reduce the rate of those who suffer from depression, as well as the suicide rate in Canada, simply by building strong communities. For example, a recent study in Italy showed that suicide rates for seniors dropped simply by having volunteers make regular phone calls to them.

As I look about my own congregation at Siloam, where I have served for the past ten years, I am again and again struck by the number of members who place notices in our weekly church bulletins, thanking people for the phone calls they received while they were off sick or struggling to cope with the death of a loved one. Many of them tell me that these phone calls from members of the congregation kept them going when they felt like giving up. Moreover, they were every bit as important as the visits they received from the trained clergy. I am also heartened by the new members of retirement age who have come to me and said, "Sheila, I can't tell you how much we are enjoying our time at Siloam. We love all the people and activities here. We feel so

---

73   Ibid.

welcome and so fulfilled!" One woman said to me, "I am so happy my husband and I found Siloam. I have a wonderful choir in which to sing, and my husband has really come alive again since you asked him to help lead the study groups. Now he is able to use his teaching gifts again."

The church is one of the few places people can make friends across the generations, where they can exercise their gifts and talents in retirement, and find spiritual nurture and guidance all in the same place. We are particularly blessed at Siloam to have a warm, caring group of people that functions more like a family rather than an organization. Like all families, we have our disagreements, but we work well together and play well together, too. Most of all, we pray and worship together, and this has made all the difference. Admittedly, not all congregations are created equal, but all congregations have the potential to be made better through our gifts of love and caring. Churches that really value their members will provide them with opportunities to use their gifts in service to others. As spiritual gerontologist Dr. Richard Johnson says, congregations "must lose the buses, bingo, and brownies attitude"[74] and encourage people to share their gifts in ways that are both productive and life-giving. Likewise, if we want to practise and maintain good mental health for the whole of our life, we will remember the wisdom of Jesus's words when he said, "Give, and it will be given to you" (Luke 6:38). Find a faith home where you can share your gifts and talents, and you will be pleasantly surprised at how much comes back to you!

---

74   Richard P. Johnson, PhD., "Shaping a New vision of Faith Formation for Maturing Adults: Sixteen Fundamental Tasks," *Lifelong Faith*, Spring 2007, 41.

In addition to finding a nurturing and caring faith home, it is also imperative that you get together with friends and others on a regular basis in the wider community. Canadian author and psychologist Susan Pinker argues that such gatherings are critical to our health and well-being, especially as we age. Indeed, the lack of close personal friendships may shorten our lives faster than cigarettes, salt, sugar, and animal fat.[75] Real-time face-to-face contact, can help us to live healthier and longer lives. Chatting with friends on the porch or over the back fence, playing cards once a week, meeting friends every Tuesday morning at the coffee shop, having friends over to dinner regularly, or going to choir practice every week, can actually lengthen your life and bring you more happiness. And get this: study after study shows that these kinds of activities will do far more to promote health and longevity than "slathering on the sunscreen, downing fistfuls of vitamins, practicing mindfulness meditation, or sweating it out at the gym or with hot yoga."[76] So, don't believe Sartre when he said, "Hell is other people."[77]

Dr. Laura L. Carstensen has made similar findings. Professor of psychology and public policy at Stanford University, Carstensen is the founding director of the Stanford Centre on Longevity. She says that we are living in an unprecedented time in human history and because of this we need to find ways to help people live longer lives that are healthier. Knowing that there are people who care about you, she observes, is essential to healthy aging. As she writes, "The perception

---

75   Susan Pinker, *The Village Effect. How Face-to-Face Contact Can Make Us Healthier and Happier.* (Toronto, Vintage Canada, 2015.), p. 7.

76   Ibid.

77   Jean-Paul Sartre, *No Exit*, 1943.

that you are alone is as great a risk factor for mortality as cigarette smoking."[78] Carstensen's observations, however, are alarming when we consider the baby-boom generation. In her observations below, Carstensen affirms what Robert Putnam noticed over fifteen years ago in his groundbreaking book, *Bowling Alone: The Collapse and Revival of American Community.*

> The fifty-five-to-sixty-four-year-olds just about to join the ranks of the elderly are far less socially engaged now than their predecessors were at the same age twenty years ago. And this pattern emerged across virtually all traditional measures of social engagement: Boomers are less likely to participate in community or religious organizations than were their counterparts twenty years ago. They are less likely to be married. They talk with their neighbours less frequently. And it doesn't stop with participation in communities and neighbourhoods: boomers report fewer meaningful interactions with their spouses and partners than did previous generations, and they report weaker ties to family and friends.[79]

In the opening pages of the bible, we are reminded of our need for community and its centrality to healthy living: "The Lord God said, 'It is not good for the man to be alone. I will make a helper suitable for him'" (Genesis 2:18). I take this not so much to be a commentary

---

78   Laura L. Carstensen, "Baby Boomers Are Isolating Themselves as They Age," *Time*, May 12, 2016. See also Robert Putnam, *Bowling Alone: The Collapse and Revival of American Community* (New York: Simon and Schuster, 2001).

79   Ibid.

on men and marriage, although studies show again and again that men live longer and happier lives when they are married; rather, I see this primarily as an observation on how essential relationships—married or single, straight or gay—are for women, men and trans-gendered. Indeed, one of our greatest fears in life, from early infancy right to older adulthood, is that we will be left alone. Perhaps this is why the authors of our United Church's *A New Creed* thought that it was so important to highlight, not once but twice, that "we are not alone."[80] Healthy living means being in a relationship with God and others.

Rabbi Richard Address, the founder and director of Jewish Sacred Aging, says that we need to really "cherish these relationships."[81] Address compares the midlife years to the Israelites' experience of wandering in exile after the Exodus from Egypt. As he notes, there are many pitfalls and slips during the journey through the wilderness:

> For many boomers, now traversing a new life stage, we can easily lose faith in our own self and in our own journey, our own story. The stresses and strains of life, adult children, grandchildren, to retire or not, our own aging parents and the challenges of caregiving; all of these now normal parts too often can combine to create a feeling of loneliness or exile. It is easy to fall into that trap.[82]

On the other hand, as he notes, this new life stage offers fresh opportunities for personal growth. While the often-challenging realities noted

---

80   The United Church of Canada, *A New Creed* (1968; rev. 1980, 1995).

81   Richard F. Address, "Exile and Love," *Jewish Sacred Aging*, February 2, 2012.

82   Ibid.

above can be and are very real for most boomers, there is wisdom we can draw on that we perhaps never fully appreciated when we were young. This has to do with the importance of relationships, including family, friends, and faith communities. The latter, as he writes, "inject a sense of love into our lives. And it is this sense of love, or intimacy, or community that is the antidote to the feeling of exile or loneliness that can often overtake us."[83] His words echo Vaillant's findings after decades of research on male development and happiness in old age—namely, that "the only thing that really matters in life are your relations to other people."[84]

As we struggle to put some temporary structures in place, or seek some shelter when the house we call life has come tumbling down around us, we do well to look to the important relationships that have sustained us in the past. A word of caution, however, is in order. To maintain these important relationships, especially relationships with children who may now live on the other side of the country, Mellinger says that we need to be prepared to take some risks.[85] This means learning new ways to stay connected through social media. While many boomers are comfortable with emailing and Facebook, not all have caught on to Skyping. The question that Mellinger often asks people is: "What risks are you willing to take in order to maintain your community?" My husband's parents in Scotland are fine people who care deeply for their children and grandchildren, but because of their fear of computers, they lost a major chance to stay connected to their grandchildren

83   Ibid.

84   George E. Vaillant, *Triumphs of Experience: The Men of the Harvard Grant Study* (Cambridge: The Belknap Press of Harvard University Press, 2012), 27.

85   Marianne Mellinger interview.

here in Canada and elsewhere in the UK, and consequently missed getting to really know them. Contrast this fear of risk-taking with a far more elderly woman in my congregation at Siloam, who lived into her hundredth year. Zena learned to use a computer and the internet at the age of ninety-seven, so that she could stay connected with her nephew, who had moved to California.

Zena also stayed very involved in her church. Here I want to emphasize that paramount among the important, life-giving relationships we enjoy in the second half of life are those that we nurture in our community of faith. Perhaps this is why I have noticed a real surge in recent years in the number of men and women in their fifties and sixties returning to church. Maybe we are now at a stage in life where the truth of Rabbi Address's words are beginning to make good sense. As he writes, our communities of faith can "provide us with a sense of direction, purpose, and soul. They lead us from exile to meaning."[86]

The Parable of the Talents

In Matthew 25:14–30, Jesus tells the famous Parable of the Talents. The story centres around a rich businessman who entrusts his money to his servants. He gives five talents (a large sum of money worth about twenty years' earnings for a labourer) to the first servant, two talents to the second, and one talent to the third. The first two servants invest the money wisely and earn 100% returns on their investments, but the third servant is afraid, and so he buries his money in the ground. When their employer returns, he praises the first two servants but shows nothing but contempt for the third servant. Of course, the story is not really about money. The point is that God has given each person gifts and talents, and God expects us to

---

86   Address, Ibid., "Exile and Love."

use them in God's service. We do not all receive the same kind or number of gifts, but we are all gifted. Since the gifts we receive are for the whole of life, it is not acceptable to simply hide them away in a closet or ignore them because we may have retired. The skills, abilities, talents, family connections, social positions, education, wisdom, and rich experiences of life must not be wasted, but need to be invested wisely at every stage of life. Sadly, like the third servant in the parable, we often fail to use our gifts to the full because we are afraid of failure. But nothing ventured, nothing gained, as the saying goes. God does not call us to be successful, only to be faithful.

One of the important gifts we receive in the second half of life is the gift of time. Again and again, I hear retired people say that they have lots of things with which to "fill their time." It makes me want to scream. This precious gift is not about filling in time. It's about making time for service, for prayer and meditation and worship. Since we need to look after the treasure that is our life, it is also about self-care. Having a wise investment plan for this period of our lives keeps us faithful and accountable and brings our lives wholeness.

Invest Wisely: Design Your Social Portfolio

The late Gene D. Cohen, a gerontologist at George Washington University, came up with a simple but brilliant concept to help all of us stay engaged with life as we age. But to make it work, we need to get started before we are truly aged. In general, people of retirement age are in the ideal position to implement it. The concept is the "social portfolio,"[87] and it looks something like this:

---

87   Gene D. Cohen, *The Creative Age. Awakening Human Potential in the Second Half of Life* (New York: Quill, Harper Collins, 2001), 265.

Gene D. Cohen's Social Portfolio

	Group Efforts	Individual Efforts
High Mobility/ High Energy	*Your activities list*	*Your activities list*
Low Mobility/ Low Energy	*Your activities list*	*Your activities list*

What does this mean? Simply put, you can think of your activities much the way you think of your financial investments. A savvy investor plans a financial portfolio with four things in mind: liquidity, diversification, emergency funds, and long-term growth. Just as you are wise to diversify your investments into different classes, so, too, are you wise to diversify your activities and interests into different classes. The reason for diversification is similar to an investment portfolio as well: some of your activities can go badly over time, much as some of your investments can. Think of the social portfolio as a kind of "insurance" in the form of vital activities that can be engaged in even in the face of disability or loss.

The same four concepts that make a good financial portfolio apply to our lifetime investments in relationships and activities. As you read the following, note also that a sound social portfolio balances *individual* with *group activities, high-energy* with *low-energy* endeavours, and *high-mobility* with *low-mobility* activities[88]:

1.   You need to have *liquidity*—hobbies, interests, and relationships to which you can easily gain access. These might include gardening, woodworking, painting, photography, cooking, reading, playing the piano, researching your family history, meditation—things that you may enjoy doing on your own. They may also include book clubs, choirs, theatre groups, walking groups, golf, curling, playing bridge, helping at a soup kitchen, working at the food bank, serving in a local service club or on a church committee—things you enjoy doing with others. Some of these activities require more physical energy while others require less. I have some boomer friends who play ice hockey every Sunday morning before church. I have another friend whose struggles with arthritis do not allow her to exercise or garden the way she used to do. Now she plants box gardens and does water-walking at the local YM-YWCA.

2.   You need to have *diversification* because circumstances may change unexpectedly.

3.   You need to have *alternative resources*—emergency funds—with which to express your creative self, if you suffer a physical decline or suffer the loss of a loved one with whom you shared social experiences.

---

88   Ibid.

4.   Finally, you need to think about the *long-term growth* of your
      creative potential through the years.[89]

Putting together an effective social portfolio takes time and thought.
For this reason, Cohen recommended that it should be done with
others who know you well. It needs to be noted, too, that one size
does not fit all. Extroverts may find it more challenging to engage in
solo activities, but having hobbies you can pursue on your own can
ease the disappointment that comes when an important social event is
cancelled due to inclement weather. More importantly, they can also
be richly rewarding. On the other hand, introverts (and only twenty-
five percent of us are true introverts[90]) may find it more challenging to
engage in regular social gatherings. Their social portfolios may include
fewer large group activities and involve only a few close friends. But as
Susan Pinker points out, "being human, introverts still need people."[91]
Indeed, their very health depends on it. As she notes, "the evidence
tells us that introverts have a greater risk of dying from cancer, and
even an increased susceptibility to catching colds, if they hunker
down alone."[92]

Just as many of us need to force ourselves to build in time for physical
exercise, so also must those of us who are more introverted make a real
effort to spend time with others. Moreover, one social outlet is not
enough. As Pinker writes:

---

89   Ibid.

90   Susan Pinker, *The Village Effect. How Face-to-Face Contact Can Make Us
      Healthier and Happier.* (Toronto, Vintage Press, 2014), p. 292.

91   Ibid.

92   Ibid.

> You may be married to the person of your dreams. But if he or she is the only person you feel close to and confide in, you're one person away from having no one at all. Immunologically speaking, you're almost naked.[93]

I saw this happen with my father when my mother died. She was really his only social contact, and because of this, his already intense grief was greatly compounded. He eventually just faded away. The only time I saw his face light up again was during a brief stay in hospital. Although he had private coverage, the only bed that was available was in the ward. Dad loved it because he finally had other people with whom to converse. When a private room eventually became available, it was no surprise to my brother and me that he declined it. In retrospect, it might have been better for him to sell his home and move into communal housing. For example, Pinker recounts the story of Bob Finn, who deliberately chose to buy a townhouse in Pleasant Hill precisely because of his more introverted nature. As he told Pinker, "At some point someone did some personality tests [of cohousing residents] and discovered that the overwhelming majority of us are introverts. Extroverts make friends anywhere. But introverts need the help of structure."[94]

While making time for group activities is necessary for good health and well-being, it is important to aim for balance in your life. That's what the social portfolio helps you achieve.

---

93   Pinker, p. 291.
94   Ibid., p. 292.

It is also in many ways a very Christ-centred approach to life. Even a casual read of the gospels reveals that Jesus understood the need for diversity and balance in life. There were many times, as when he preached to crowds by the sea of Galilee or on the mountaintop, or when he fed the multitudes, where his journey took him into large group situations, demanding high personal energy. Even just *getting to* the mountaintop involved some major hill climbing! There were other occasions, as when he sat by a well, ministering to the Samaritan woman, or when he reclined at a table with his dear friends Mary, Martha, and Lazarus, that he found himself in smaller and more intimate settings. Then there was the ongoing, day-to-day training of his often dunderheaded disciples, whose frequent bickering and jostling for places of privilege must surely have required a major investment of time and emotional energy, not to mention a full itinerary in terms of teaching and travel. Yet in Luke's Gospel, we learn that Jesus was also in the habit of taking time to be by himself: "But Jesus Himself would often slip away to the wilderness and pray" (Luke 6:15, NASB). Being a disciple of Jesus means balancing individual with group activities and high-energy with low-energy endeavours, as well as high-mobility with low-mobility interests. And interspersed among all these activities, we need to set aside time with God in prayer.

Living in the In-Between Time

> In the first book, Theophilus, I wrote about all that Jesus did and taught from the beginning 2 until the day when he was taken up to heaven, after giving instructions through the Holy Spirit to the apostles whom he had chosen. 3 After his suffering he presented himself alive to them by many convincing proofs, appearing to them during forty days

and speaking about the kingdom of God. ⁴ *While eating with them, he ordered them not to leave Jerusalem, but to wait there for the promise of the Father. "This," he said, "is what you have heard from me;* ⁵ *for John baptized with water, but you will be baptized with the Holy Spirit not many days from now."*

⁶ *So when they had come together, they asked him, "Lord, is this the time when you will restore the kingdom to Israel?"* ⁷ *He replied, "It is not for you to know the times or periods that the Father has set by his own authority.* ⁸ *But you will receive power when the Holy Spirit has come upon you; and you will be my witnesses in Jerusalem, in all Judea and Samaria, and to the ends of the earth."* ⁹ *When he had said this, as they were watching, he was lifted up, and a cloud took him out of their sight.* ¹⁰ *While he was going and they were gazing up toward heaven, suddenly two men in white robes stood by them.* ¹¹ *They said, "Men of Galilee, why do you stand looking up toward heaven? This Jesus, who has been taken up from you into heaven, will come in the same way as you saw him go into heaven."*

¹² *Then they returned to Jerusalem from the mount called Olivet, which is near Jerusalem, a Sabbath day's journey away.* ¹³ *When they had entered the city, they went to the room upstairs where they were staying, Peter, and John, and James, and Andrew, Philip, and Thomas, Bartholomew and Matthew, James son of Alphaeus, and Simon the Zealot, and Judas son of James.* ¹⁴ *All these were constantly devoting themselves to prayer, together with*

*certain women, including Mary the mother of Jesus, as
well as his brothers.*

– Acts 1:1–14

One of the best examples of how people cope during the confusing
and bewildering time of the Neutral Zone comes from the Book of
Acts (Acts 1:1–14). The author paints for us a very sad story, a story
about saying goodbye. You will remember that after the Resurrection,
Jesus stayed with his disciples and continued to teach them for forty
days. Then, after he had completed his instructions, "he was taken up
before their very eyes, and a cloud hid him from their sight." And so,
Luke tells us, "The disciples returned to Jerusalem from the hill called
the Mount of Olives, a Sabbath day's walk from the city."

Luke doesn't actually tell us how they were feeling. He doesn't have
to. We can well imagine that their mood must have been one of deep
sorrow as they watched Jesus being taken from their sight. This is a
shattered community. They have lost their leader. Worse, they have lost
their best friend.

And so, they don't know what to do. They remember some words of
Jesus and they go to the upper room to try and figure things out, and
to hope that his words might come true and something might happen.
But for the moment they find themselves in a state of shock, a kind of
limbo. They are in the Neutral Zone, living in the "in-between time,"
between loss and promise. In the Church year, we would say that they
are between the Ascension and Pentecost, between the departure of
Jesus and the coming of the Spirit. But what's really going on is that
the disciples no longer know who they really are. Their beloved leader
is gone. What do they do now? Go back to their jobs as fishermen?

And what about Matthew? He can hardly return to his former career as a tax collector. Without Jesus, who are they? How are they supposed to act now?

Luke tells us that the first thing they did was to pray. Remember, it was a very difficult time for them. Their beloved leader was dead, and while he had promised them the gift of the Spirit, this had not yet happened. They didn't know whether they had a future as a sect or as a religion, or whether they should just split up and go back into the mainstream. So, they sought solace by joining together in prayer.

Note that the scripture story says that they joined "together" in prayer. They came together as a community. In the end, all genuine experiences of aloneness lead us back into community. We may need to spend a good length of time on our own in the wilderness, but, inevitably, we return to our metaphorical village to share the wisdom we have learned in solitude.

Communities, while never perfect, can provide innumerable benefits. Developing good friendships will also be important in the retirement period. Research has shown, for example, that friendship:

- increases your sense of belonging and purpose;

- boosts your happiness;

- reduces stress;

- improves your self-worth;

- decreases your risk of serious mental illness;

- helps you weather traumas, such as divorce, serious illness, job loss, and the death of loved ones;

- encourages you to change unhealthy lifestyle habits, such as excessive drinking or lack of exercise;

- helps you celebrate your good times, with the offer of comfort during the bad.[95]

There is no question that good friendships take work, especially in the post-retirement period when it is not as easy to make friends through your work or through the Home and School Association or Little League baseball. But developing new hobbies, participating in your church or house of faith, or getting involved with other organizations, can bring new friendships and a sense of community.

The disciples had given up jobs and families to follow Jesus. It was only natural, therefore, when Jesus was taken from them, that their first reaction was to seek comfort and solace in one another's company. That's what friends do. They come together to support one another through major life transitions, to pray for each other during dark nights of fear and illness and sorrow, and to help one another navigate times of confusion and chaos when the home that is our life appears to be in shambles.

For Further Reading:

Anne Beattie-Stokes, *A Heart of Wisdom. Inspiration and Instruction for Conscious Elderhood.* (Booksurge Publishing, 2009)

---

95   Mayo Clinic, *Friendships: Enrich your life and improve your health, Discover the connection between health and friendship, and how to promote and maintain healthy friendships*, June 9, 2011.

Gene D. Cohen, *The Creative Age. Awakening Human Potential in the Second Half of Life.* (New York: Quill, Harper Collins, 2001.)

Richard F. Address, *Seekers of Meaning. Baby Boomers, Judaism, and the Pursuit of Healthy Aging.* (New York, URJ Press, 2012.)

For Viewing:

Amour. Michael Haneke, Director, 2012. An octogenarian couple's bond of love is severely tested when the wife suffers a stroke.

Hope Springs. Directed by David Frankel. 2012.

Re-Designing Your Life: A Practical Spirituality for the Second Half of Life, Sheila Macdonald Macgregor, Wib Dawson, videographer and editor, 2017.

Questions for Discussion:

Watch Session Three of the videos that have been made to accompany this book and then discuss the following. Note: if you are leading a study group, you may not have time to discuss all the questions. Choose those that you feel will be most helpful to your group.

1. Bridges says that time in the Neutral Zone can be very lonely and chaotic, and yet it is also the period during which the true work of transformation takes place. Using coloured pencils, markers, or crayons, create a picture that represents how you felt when you found yourself living through a time

of chaos and confusion. You may also create a collage from magazines and newspapers that convey how you felt.[96]

2.   Group Exercise: Depending on your responses to the following, stand on the right or left side of the room. You may also choose to stand in the middle of the room if you like both options equally:

You have a free evening. (1) You spend it with friends (right side of room). (2) You would prefer to stay home and read a book (left side of room).

You have a chance to travel. You decide (1) to go on a cruise or a bus tour so that you can mix with and meet new people (right side). (2) You choose to go to a cabin the woods or a silent retreat (left side).

On your afternoon off, you choose to (1) play golf (right side) or (2) work in your garden (left side).

Friday nights you (1) love to go to the theatre with friends (right side) or (2) stay home and watch the hockey game with a good friend (left side).

Think of some other examples that you can add to this ice-breaker. Have fun!

3.   Read Exodus 3:4–6. How was Moses's life transformed in the wilderness? Compare with the story of Jesus in the wilderness

---

96   My thanks to United Church of Canada Diaconal Ministry Candidate Barbara McGill for this and other suggestions on how to use the creative arts to explore meaning in the second half of life.

in Matthew 4:1–11. Now consider the significance of community for Christians.

4. Anne Beattie-Stokes found her calling while on a wilderness retreat. Reflect upon those times in your own life when you have either gone on a personal retreat, or withdrawn from your usual round of activities to mediate and pray. How did these times away help you to discern the call of God's Spirit? Why is it important for Christians to withdraw for times of reflection and prayer?

5. Read Genesis 2:18. Reflect also on the United Church of Canada's *A New Creed*. Why is it so important for Christians to stay engaged in a faith community? How would you respond to the person who asserts that he or she can be a Christian without participating in a local congregation?

6. Read Matthew 25:14–30. How is Christ calling you to use your God-given talents and gifts in service to others and the building up of God's Kingdom? What happens, according to the parable, when we fail to use our gifts to the full?

7. Name some examples from the gospels that reveal that Jesus knew the importance of balancing high-energy activities with low-energy activities, high-mobility activities with low-mobility events, and individual times of prayer with group worship and activities. Using the example of Jesus, and the model provided by Cohen, put together your own social portfolio. Think about your natural tendencies and how you might balance out your profile. (How might you develop new friendships and community? How might you find quiet

space?) Share with one or two close friends who know you well and get their feedback.

8. Read Acts 1:1–14. What is the first thing the disciples do after their beloved friend and Lord ascends to heaven? What can we learn from their actions to help us in our times of loneliness and confusion? When caring for an elderly parent or partner? When suffering from grief?

9. What are some things you can do to strengthen existing relationships and foster new friendships in retirement? Where will you find support for your journey in retirement or when the kids leave home? How do you think discerning your call and making changes affect your family and friends? As a group, name some strategies that might help you stay focused and live into God's call.

10. What do you need to discuss with your partner before you or they retire? With your elderly parents? With your adult children?

11. Reflecting on Bill and Karen Butt's experience when they told friends about their intention to serve the church in Mozambique, how can well-meaning friends undermine or hinder God's call on our lives? How do we stay alert to where God is calling us to serve?

12. If you have time, arrange to meet up again to view *Amour* or *Hope Springs*. What do we learn from the characters in these films about the challenges that couples in long-term

relationships often face and how we can find ways to renew our love in the second half of life?

Chapter 4:
Still Renovating!

One of the first things you discover when you undertake home renovations is that they always take far longer than you imagined they would, so you should not be surprised that we are still talking about renovations.

In our last chapter, we noted how essential it is to take time in the Neutral Zone, that place of pandemonium where our house lies in ruins, and where there is no clear path forward. However painful and challenging life may be for us with the rubble of demolished walls, the period of rebuilding can be just as turbulent and confusing. Whether we are undergoing the end of an important relationship or saying farewell to a career that brought our life purpose and meaning, this is a chaotic and often bewildering time. Yet it is paramount that we do not rush this period because this is the stage in which we are at our most creative. Taking the time we need to reflect on what we want to do next, and where and how God is calling us to live our life in the future, will reap huge personal benefits. A good carpenter or licensed architect, for example, spends hours visiting and analyzing the building site and gathering information from the clients about their design ideas, budget, and housing needs before the final written plan is ever presented. If a well-thought-out plan is essential to the successful completion of a building project, consider how much more it is needed when trying to rebuild the house that is your life.

The River of Life

A good renovation plan is like a good map. It shows you the basic footprint of your existing house (or what's left of it) and where you've been, and it lays out a picture of what you hope to achieve and where you want to go next. One of the exercises Bridges invited people to consider as they were trying to figure out where they'd been and where they wanted to head next was a map called "the River Named 'You.'"[97] In this exercise, he encouraged people to see their lives as a river. Then he asked them to consider where their headwaters were, the sources that influenced them in life. Next, he asked them to describe the country into which the river of their life drains. Is it flat or mountainous? Is it a desert wilderness or is it a major metropolis? Is the river shallow or deep? Is it slow and graceful, or full of fast-paced, heart-stopping rapids and beautiful but dangerous waterfalls? After mapping out all these things on their river, they were asked to include details about the kind of traffic they found along their river, noting the exports and imports of their river basin as well.

In the summer of 2016, I had an opportunity to really live with this metaphor for a weekend as my husband and I travelled by boat with my cousins Craig and Doris Macdonald down the French River, often considered the dividing line between northern and southern Ontario. Designated a Canadian Heritage River in 1985, the French River was used as a transportation corridor by the Algonquin peoples who lived in this region. The Ojibwas people named it the "French River" because

---

97   Bridges, *The Way of Transition*, 89–90.

of the early French explorers and missionaries who navigated its waters back in the seventeenth century. Those who travelled this waterway included explorers like Étienne Brûlé, Samuel de Champlain, Pierre-Esprit Radisson, and, later, Scottish and English explorers like Simon Fraser, Alexander Mackenzie, and David Thompson.

Beautiful, rugged, and awe-inspiring, this journey was much more than a picturesque trip down the river. It also represented a search for my roots. My maternal great-grandfather Crombie settled in one of the inlets, now known as Crombie's Bay, back in the second half of the nineteenth century. He spent months of back-breaking work clearing one of the few tracts of arable land in this rocky terrain so that it would be suitable to farm. It was here that his son Ellis, my Grandpa Crombie, grew up and learned to navigate the river in all kinds of weather. As a boy, he loved to shoot the rapids. Like his father before him, when he got a bit older, Ellis ran the mail boat that stopped at all the small settlements along the river. Here, also, he would portage around the rapids while pulling a heavy load of mail behind him or, in the winter, travel by dogsled across the frozen river. Here he would pick the wild blueberries that he loved so much and that grew in the woods. Here, too, he would later pick the water lilies that composed the bouquet for his young bride, newly arrived from Ireland.

How my Irish grandmother ever survived in that breathtaking but also desolate wilderness, I cannot even begin to conceive. Arriving just before winter set in back in 1904, I can imagine how she must have longed for the familiar sights and sounds of the big, bustling city of Dublin she had left, not to mention her family and friends across the ocean. However, she was soon to face an even greater challenge than a portage around the rapids and the starkness of heavy forest and rugged glaciated rock. The half-uncle who had promised her and her siblings an exciting adventure in the New World neglected to inform them of the dangers of the logging industry to which her brothers would be subjected or the fact that she and her sister would be expected to provide entertainment to the men at the logging camp. It was quite a shock to this pious young woman and her family. My grandfather, Ellis Crombie, obviously realised that they had no idea what they were getting themselves into and told them that they could always board at his mother's home if they changed their minds about living with their uncle. It was not long before my grandmother got word to the Crombies that she and her sister needed to find another place to lodge. The story is that as soon as their uncle went off to the logging camp one morning, the two women waited silently with bags packed by the front door, making a mad dash for my grandfather's sleigh as soon as they heard his horses' sleigh bells. My grandmother never returned to Ireland to live. She married Ellis Crombie the following spring, carrying as her wedding bouquet the lilies that he had picked that morning on the French River.

That was well over a hundred years ago. While the farm is no more, the rustic beauty of the French River continues to draw many tourists and cottagers who seek a peaceful escape from their busy urban lives and demanding schedules. There is lots to explore. The river is really a series of island-dotted lakes connected by rapids and falls that gently lower the river a total of sixty feet from Lake Nipissing to Georgian Bay.

As I was reflecting on our trip down the French River, I now understood why Bridges compares our life to a river, for our lives are indeed very much like a river. There are the strong headwaters—the parents and teachers who first introduced us to the faith and helped to shape us into the people we are today. There is the surrounding country into which the river of our life drains, touching the lives of those we encounter along life's way. There are days when all seems well, and our river flows lazily and peacefully through the beautiful countryside, and then there are days when the terrain becomes rocky, and we encounter fast-paced and treacherous rapids. There is the traffic we find along our river, the friends we import into our river basin as we journey and also the exports, the ones to whom we must sadly say goodbye as our river travels ever closer to the sea of eternity. Throughout it all, there is the hand of God, guiding and supporting us along our way.

As I think back over my own life, I see strong headwaters in my parents, special teachers, and the people who formed my "church" or "faith home"—friends and mentors in the United Church, in which I was baptized, confirmed, married, and ordained, but also friends across denominational lines: my Baptist friend Elizabeth and her mother, who was one of my leaders in the Pioneer Girls group to which I belonged as a young girl, in addition to the United Church Explorers group at my home church; my history professor at the University of Windsor, a Roman Catholic brother by the name of Brother Bonaventure Miner, who was the first person to ever really listen to my thoughts; and, as well, the professors who opened up the riches of the scriptures and Christian theology to me at two Presbyterian colleges—Princeton and, later, McCormick Theological Seminary in Chicago, as well as in my year as a ministerial assistant at Liberton Kirk in Edinburgh.

I can identify places where my river ambled gently and happily through lush countryside, the satisfaction brought by marriage to a supremely good, kind, and patient man. There have been exciting moments, as when our four children came into our lives. But there have also been times, before and since, when my life seemed to enter a bleak wilderness, bereft of the friends who brought my life meaning. Like most people who reach the second half of life, I have had my fair share of imports and exports, as I am continually blessed by new friends, while at the same time saddened by how I have lost touch with old friends and suffered the deaths of others. There has also been the joy of serving seven different congregations in the United Church of Canada, as well as the normal ups and downs that go with congregational life.

If I look carefully at my life, I notice a theme emerging. All my life, I have been a student, whether formally or informally. When I returned to school a few years ago, to undertake research for my Doctor of Ministry degree, my eldest sons, Lachlan and John, were shocked to learn that this was not a requirement laid on by my congregation. They couldn't believe that I would want to go back to school in my mid-fifties! To those who have known me all my life, this was no surprise. In my ministry, it has been the teaching and learning aspects of my call that have spoken most deeply to me. I am not an intellectual, nor am I a dilettante. I am just someone who loves to learn new things, whether in the university classroom or the classroom of life. My learning has been made possible because of encouraging parents and teachers, a loving and supportive husband, and the wonderful congregations I have served—not to mention, more formally, by the generous support of the United Church of Canada Foundation. I have been truly blessed.

Vocation and Calling Versus Job and Occupation

As you reflect upon the various twists and turns your life has taken, you may begin to see a pattern. You may notice a theme emerging.

Pay special attention to this, as it may help you to understand your life's calling.

Christians believe that everyone has a God-given calling. Our calling, according to the Apostle Paul, is stated in the fourth chapter of his first letter to the Corinthian church. "Think of us this way, as servants of Christ and stewards of God's mysteries." (1 Corinthians 4:1). Paul believed that all work has sacred meaning. In chapter 12 of his *First Letter to the Corinthians*, Paul writes: "There are many ways of serving, but the same God is served. There are different abilities to perform service, but the same God gives ability to each of us. The Spirit's presence is shown in some way in each person for the good of all" (1 Corinthians 12:5 GNV).

The great Protestant reformer Martin Luther used to say that "vocation" is "the mask of God."[98] It's how God works in the world, in and through all of us. As Teresa of Avila once said, "Christ has no body now but yours. No hands, no feet on earth but yours. Yours are the eyes through which he looks compassion on this world. Yours are the feet with which he walks to do good. Yours are the hands through which he blesses all the world. Yours are the hands, yours are the feet, yours are the eyes, you are his body. Christ has no body now on earth but yours."

Too often, however, we tend to confuse our job with our vocation. So, let's be clear: *our call or vocation is not our employment history.* It's not our job resumé. There are often connections between what we did in our work life and how we have felt called to serve God, then and now. But our vocation does not end when we retire. I like the way Clayton

---

98   Gene Edward Veith Jr., *God at Work* (Wheaton, IL: Cressway, 2002), 24.

defines vocation. He says that vocation "is rather the core thread around which one's various jobs or activities are often wrapped."[99]

Ironically, it is often clergy who have the greatest trouble distinguishing their call to serve God with the call to serve in a particular ministry job in a congregation. Clayton found that the women and men who had the most difficulty understanding this distinction were those who had spent their whole lives in ministry to the church. In reflecting on his work with clergy in retirement, Clayton tells a story about a colleague. After she retired from her many years as an ordained minister, she turned to him and said: "Who am I now that I am not working? If I have no job, then I have no calling."[100] The problem was not that her years working in the ministry of the church was not a calling. It was. The problem was that she had confused the public role of minister with her call and could not see that in fact her calling was to the whole of life, regardless of whether or not she was employed by a congregation.

But of course, clergy are not the only people who fail to recognize that our calling is much larger than a job or occupation. Clayton says that this is just the first of several false assumptions people make about their call or vocation.

Common Misunderstandings about Vocation

It is interesting here to pause and consider what we mean by the word "vocation" and how its meaning has changed through the centuries. Many people today think that to be called is to be employed. But this was not always how the word was understood.

---

99   Clayton, *Called for Life*, 7.

100   Ibid., 1.

The word vocation comes from the Latin word *vocare*, which, in Latin, means "to call." In the New Testament, Jesus called his disciples to follow. He promised no employment, no job, no occupation. They were simply invited to be disciples, followers, learners.

Over the centuries, the meaning of the word vocation changed. The church linked the calling of the disciples to the role of the clergy or those in religious orders. The Protestant Reformation changed this, expanding the understanding of vocation to include lay people, as well.

However, over time, the term vocation was changed again by common usage so that most people came to equate "calling" with "employment." Clayton writes that somehow, we need to recover the original meaning of the phrase "called by God."[101] To be called is to follow in the way, not to have a specific job or profession. When the job comes to an end, you still have a calling, a vocation.

A second false assumption that people often make, says Clayton, is to assume that to be called is to have had a profound spiritual experience.[102] While it is often true that a calling involves a spiritual experience, it is much more often the case that God speaks to us through a kindly aunt, teacher, friend, parent, or even a stranger.

I am reminded now of the delightful story that Father William Bausch told of a woman who was in great distress because she had lost the sense of God in her life. "Why don't I feel God's presence? If only I could feel God or know that God had touched me."

---

101   Ibid., 7.

102   Ibid., 8.

The woman to whom she was complaining said to her, "Pray to God. Ask God to touch you, and you will feel God's hand touching you."

So, the woman closed her eyes and began to pray in earnest—and suddenly she felt the hand of God touching her! She cried out, "God touched me!" and went into an ecstasy of joy. But then she paused and said, "But you know, it felt just like your hand."

And the other woman replied, "Of course it did. It was my hand."

"It was?"

"Of course, what did you think God would be doing? Did you think God would extend a long arm out of heaven to touch you? God just took the hand that was nearest and used that."[103]

Jesus has promised us the gift of the Spirit, but the Spirit comes to meet us most often not in the burning bush, but in the hand of a friend. Indeed, as Jesus promised, "wherever two or three are gathered together, there am I in the midst of them" (Matthew: 18:20 KJV).

At other times, God may speak to us through an event or series of events that occurred in our life that result in a kind of epiphany or some new insight. Secondly, when we are called, this does not mean that we are "like puppets at the end of a string."[104] God still expects us to make decisions, set goals, and be accountable for our actions.

---

103   William J. Bausch, *60 More Seasonal Homilies* (Mystic, CT: Twenty-Third Publications, 2002), 171.

104   Clayton, *Called for Life*, p. 8.

A third false assumption that Clayton identifies is to assume that to be called is to have a single direction in life.[105] Once a plumber, always a plumber, or once a teacher, always a teacher. You may well continue some aspects of your former job, especially if you loved your work. For example, the plumber may decide to donate his time in retirement to helping build homes for Habitat for Humanity. Or she may decide that she really wants to pursue her love of gardening and help out at a community garden. Likewise, the teacher may volunteer to lead one of the study groups at the church or tutor refugee children at the local library or community centre. Or he may wish to try something completely new like photography and volunteer to take photos for the monthly church newsletter or the local wildlife gazette.

The famous scientist William Lawrence Bragg, a physicist and X-ray specialist, is still the youngest person ever to have received the Nobel Prize. He was only twenty-five. When he left his teaching position at the University of Cambridge and moved to London, he missed having a garden and so worked as a part-time gardener, unrecognized by his employer, until a guest at the house expressed surprise at seeing him there. Apparently, he would just wander the streets until he found a garden that looked interesting and had potential and then he would ask the owner if he could do the gardening. You can imagine the home-owners' surprise at learning that their gardener was a world-famous scientist and Nobel Prize winner!

Unfortunately, not many of us are like Bragg. Far too often, we feel locked for life into one task, but we need to remember that Jesus himself did not have a single calling. As a young man, he was called to

---

105   Ibid., pp. 8-9.

serve in the family carpentry shop. Then, at the age of thirty, he was baptized in the River Jordan, sent out into the desert by the Spirit, and emerged with a new calling to share the love of God with God's people. No doubt he shared his love of God even as he worked as a carpenter; but now his calling took on a new shape and form, for now he would be going out to teach and preach the Good News on a full-time basis.

Likewise, the disciples' calling underwent more than one transformation. The disciples were called first to be followers and learners. Then, with the death and resurrection of Jesus, they were to be leaders, teachers, preachers, and healers—the embodiment of Christ himself. As Clayton observes, although they were called to follow Jesus, their role changed over the years and with the changing circumstances.[106] Thus, within our calling, too, is the requirement to be open to change.

I like the way my friend Bill Butt describes it. He says that at various places along his life's journey, he has been called "to reinvent himself".[107] God's call is for the whole of his life, but how he lives out that call at any given time is open to change.

It's interesting to note, by the way, just when it was that the disciples received their call to follow Jesus. All of them were already established in careers, which means that they were likely men of a somewhat more mature age. Consider Jesus himself. When he experienced his call to teach and preach, he was already around thirty years old. In our culture, this is still considered a young adult, but in Jesus's time, he was entering the final third of his life. We know, for example, based on the records we have of various censuses taken in Egypt during the

---

106   Ibid., p. 8.
107   Ibid., Karen and Bill Butt interview.

Roman occupation, that the average life span for men in Jesus's day was thirty-nine or forty years, and that average life span for women was thirty-four years. Given the historical context, this means that, in contemporary terms, Jesus would have been about age sixty when God called him to go out and preach the gospel. And of course, we cannot forget that Jesus's mentor, John the Baptist, was the offspring of two elderly parents—Elizabeth and Zechariah—who had almost given up hope of ever having a child.

Looking to other religious traditions, it is well to note that the Buddha was even older than Jesus was when he heard his call—probably thirty-five or older. Mohamed was forty or older when he began to teach, and Abraham and Sarah, at age seventy-five, were thought to be extremely elderly when they received God's call to travel to a new land. Likewise, Moses was very elderly when, at the age of eighty, God called him to leave behind the tending of his father-in-law's flocks and return to Egypt to lead God's people out of slavery—no small task for someone of Moses's age or, indeed, of any age! To take a more contemporary example, Winston Churchill was sixty-six when he became prime minister of Britain. So, God continues to call people to serve well after the time of midlife.

Finally, as Clayton notes, to be called does not mean that you get a set of clearly outlined God-given instructions to follow.[108] Flexibility and an openness to the Spirit's leading are needed if one is to properly discern where God is calling one to serve. In the *Book of Acts*, the disciples had no notice of what was going to happen next. Like us, they stumbled along, praying to God that they would be faithful. So, also,

---

108   Clayton, *Called for Life*, 8–9.

we must be prepared to spend time with God in prayer if we are to remain honest and steadfast.

To sum up, our call is to the *whole* journey of life, not just the first or the second part. Indeed, as Stevens points out, "even the helpful book titled 'Second Half'" may be misleading. Stevens says that such terms as "first half/second half" may give the erroneous impression that God's call is only for a particular half of life or that there is no connection between the two halves of life.[109] The call itself is to a pilgrimage that lasts our whole life long.

How to Find Your Passion

The eloquent nineteenth-century British prime minister, Benjamin Disraeli, once observed that individuals "are only great when they act from passion." Disraeli should have known. As the son of humble Jewish parents who had converted to the Christian faith, he encountered a lot of prejudice in his rise to the top of "the greasy pole" of politics, but his determination and passion finally won out. Today he is ranked among the top ten of all British prime ministers.

Chances are that if you can name that thing about which you feel passionate, you will also discover where and how God is calling you to serve. Howard Thurman, the great African American author, theologian, civil rights leader, and mentor to Martin Luther King, Jr., once said: "Don't worry about what the world needs. Ask what makes you come alive and do that, because what the world needs is people who

---

109   R. Paul Stevens, *Aging Matters: Finding your calling for the rest of your life* (Grand Rapids: William B. Eerdmann's Publishing House, 2016), 72.

have come alive."[110] In other words, what God's world needs is passionate people. The author of the *Book of Revelation* even goes so far as to proclaim that God despises our lukewarmness. "I know your works; you are neither cold nor hot. I wish that you were either cold or hot. So, because you are lukewarm, and neither cold nor hot, I am about to spit you out of my mouth" (Revelation 3:15-16).

What is Passion?

Before we look more closely at how we discover our passion in retirement, it's important to note that psychologists and counsellors tend to make a distinction between "motivation" and "passion." According to retirement coach Janet Christensen, motivation is always externally driven.[111] We can be motivated by things that are positives. The most common example of this kind of motivation is in the area of sales, where a salesperson may be working with a bonus structure and so will be motivated to work hard in order to get the bonus that comes from a sale. Motivation can also be created out of need. For example, someone who has a family to support may need to work three jobs to make ends meet. Motivation can also be externally driven by deadlines. As Christensen notes, "we're all motivated in April to get our income tax returns in, but I don't think anyone really enjoys it unless they're getting a big refund. They enjoy the refund, not necessarily the process."[112] The point is that motivation is always externally driven,

---

110 Quoted from website of BU Howard Thurman Centre for Common Ground, George Sherman Union, 775 Commonwealth Ave., Lower Level, Boston, MA 02215.

111 Janet Christensen interview.

112 Ibid.

sometimes because of very positive motives, but sometimes out of need or structure.

Passion, on the other hand, is very different. Christensen says that it happens when we have those kinds of Zen moments in which we feel so energized and passionate about what we are doing that we actually lose track of time. As she notes, the word "passion" really derives from the word "inspiration," which comes from the Latin word *inspirare*. Simply put, this means "that which comes from the spirit." The Romans believed that inspiration was the direct result of the influence of the gods. A god would "blow into" or "breathe upon" a man or woman, and thereby inflame or excite that individual to undertake some great deed. In the biblical tradition, it was God's Spirit hovering over creation that led to the birth of the cosmos in the *Book of Genesis*. Likewise, in *Genesis*, the first human being was created when "the Lord God formed man of the dust of the ground, and *breathed into* his nostrils the *breath* of life; and man became a living soul." (Genesis 2:7) It is interesting to note that the original Hebrew word that is used in this text is the word for "spirit," *ruach*, which can mean breath, wind, or spirit. It is God's spirit or breath that gives breath and life to humankind.

Many of us grew up singing the old hymn "Breathe on Me, Breath of God," which my congregation continues to find uplifting and inspiring. It was written by Edwin Hatch, an English theologian who taught classics at the University of Toronto's Trinity College, and at Morrin College in Quebec City. In the hymn, Hatch asks God to breathe (*inspirare*) new life into him so that he will have life anew and so that his heart and will may be one with God. He prays that his earthly part may glow with fire divine. This seems a very fitting hymn for those of

us entering the second half of life. As we seek out our p
that we, too, may have new life breathed into our bei
heart may not only be one with God but also on fire ol .

Finding Your Passion

So, what makes you come alive? What things are you passionate about?

First, begin by making an inventory of your talents. What are you good at? Write it down—all of it. This is no place for undue modesty. True, you may not be at the top in your field; but you still have talent. My husband, Richard, is a good golfer. He has played golf since he was a young boy growing up in St. Andrews, Scotland, where he watched many a fine golfer play the famous Old Course, including his own father, who won the Boys British Open back in 1946. Is Richard a great golfer? He would likely confess that he is not, but he does have some talent for the game and loves to play it. Likewise, you may be a fine artist. The fact that you are not and probably never will be another Tom Thomson or Emily Carr does not mean that you do not have genuine talent. So, forget the false modesty. Remember the popular bumper sticker: "God don't make no junk!" God gave you talents, too. Name them and celebrate them!

Again, remember to list everything you do well. There are things at which you may be supremely talented, but have never really considered to be a talent. For example, we have a lovely photo of our beautiful niece Rebecca when she was in the first grade of elementary school in Edinburgh. She is smiling happily and lovingly as she hugs her little kitten close to her. Some years after her mother sent us the photo, we learned that it was part of a school assignment in which each of the children was asked to name something at which they were good.

Rebecca shared the photo of her and her kitten and then announced to the class: "I am good at loving my kitty." What better talent could there be, especially in our often-troubled world! Indeed, when I consider the number of scarred and hurting people who haunt the offices of psychologists and therapists, I cannot think of a better talent to possess than to be able to love another well.

Secondly, look for your passion in your suffering. This may seem like an unusual place to look for your calling or vocation in the second half of life. Our culture today does everything it can to avoid suffering. There are even mega-church preachers and TV evangelists who have become very popular espousing a "prosperity gospel," promising riches and relief from suffering. Health, wealth, and happiness can all be yours! All you need to do is be faithful—and, of course, be generous in what you place on the offering plate! As James Goff noted in a 1990 *Christianity Today* article, the prosperity gospel reduces God "to a kind of 'cosmic bellhop', attending to the needs and desires of His creation."[113] It knows nothing of the "abundant life" which Christ promises us, an abundance that can be experienced irrespective of the circumstances of our lives and even amidst great suffering.

Life coach Christine Hassler encourages her clients to look for their passion somewhere they might not think to look: in their suffering. What does she mean by this?[114]

The original definition of the word "passion" is actually "suffering." The Passion of Christ, for example, is a reference to the sufferings of

---

113   James R. Goff, Jr., "The Faith That Claims," *Christianity Today 34* (Feb. 1990), 21.

114   Christine Hassler, Blog, November 29, 2012.

Christ between the night of the Last Supper and his death. Over time, the word passion has evolved to mean: "love; a strong liking or desire for or devotion to some activity, object, or concept."

So, the word passion means two things: suffering and love. There is key information in this. Many people who are truly doing something they are incredibly passionate about were inspired by their own suffering.

Think about Canadian reformer Tommy Douglas. Shortly before he left Scotland, Douglas fell and injured his right knee. Osteomyelitis set in, and he underwent many operations in Scotland in an attempt to cure the condition. Later, however, in Winnipeg, the osteomyelitis flared up again, and Douglas was sent to the hospital. Doctors there told his parents his leg would have to be amputated. Fortunately, a well-known orthopaedic surgeon took an interest in his case and agreed to treat the boy for free if his parents would allow medical students to observe. After several operations, Douglas's leg was saved. This experience convinced him that health care should be free to all. "I felt that no boy should have to depend either for his leg or his life upon the ability of his parents to raise enough money to bring a first-class surgeon to his bedside,"[115] Douglas told an interviewer many years later. Therein was born the dream and Douglas's passion for a system of universal health care, from which all Canadians now benefit today.

The great Canadian educational reformer and founder of the international women's organization known as the Women's Institute, Adelaide Hoodless, discovered her passion through her affliction, too. It was after she lost her precious infant son Jack at age fourteen months that

---

115   Lewis H. Thomas, ed., *The Making of a Socialist: The Recollections of T.C. Douglas* (Edmonton: University of Alberta Press, 1982), 7.

Adelaide began her public life. Jack had died from drinking contaminated milk. From then on, Adelaide's passion was to ensure that women had the knowledge to prevent deaths like that of her beloved Jack, and she devoted herself to the betterment of education for new mothers.

Pauline and Al are two of the most devoted and caring people I know. We are so blessed to have them as members at Siloam. There, they raised three beautiful and talented daughters. But tragedy struck when their middle daughter, Catherine, was killed by a drunken driver one warm summer's evening in August of 1997. They were heartbroken. Their lives were shattered. But with the support of their family, as well as their friends at Siloam, they worked hard to rebuild their lives and honour Catherine's memory through their service to Mothers Against Drunk Driving (MADD). For years, Pauline spent many hours with people who had been charged with driving under the influence of alcohol to help them understand the devastation their recklessness could cause and so change their ways. Today, Pauline and Al continue to participate in fundraisers for MADD in our city. Through their generous service and witness, they continue to be an inspiration to our congregation, our community, and especially those who have experienced intense suffering in their lives. Their story was profoundly shaped by another parent who lost a child to a drunken driver: Candy Lightener, the founder of MADD.

While none of us actively seeks sorrow or hardship, sometimes, this is where we find our passion. Looking at how we have experienced suffering in our life may be a place for us to start considering what it is we are passionate about. And if we are currently experiencing pain in our lives, we may wish to consider Dr. Jane Thibault's concept of "dedicated suffering," where we take our suffering energy and, through our prayers, dedicate it to another person (or cause) and ask God that it may be used to help this individual.

Thirdly, pay attention to who makes you annoyed or jealous. Are there people doing things that are "frivolous" who annoy you? Take a closer look at that annoyance. Is the truth behind your annoyance that you really wish you could live so freely, that you didn't have so many serious responsibilities and could be as "immature" as they are?

Dr. Susan Biali, a medical doctor, nutritionist, life coach, personal-development expert, and late-blooming flamenco dancer, says that she spent years being an overachieving and doing-what-everyone-expects-of-me student. Then, one day, she decided to embark on what she calls her "Mexican adventure" to give herself a break and find time to pursue her passions for writing and dancing. Most people thought she was nuts, but her father got the angriest. He told her that she was wasting her life and should let him help her set up her own medical clinic, instead.[116]

He pounded the kitchen table with his fist, shouting, "Life isn't supposed to be fun! When are you going to grow up like the rest of us?" She ignored him, as she did everyone else who tried to discourage her.

A few years later, when it was clear that living, writing, and dancing in Mexico was one of the best decisions (and career moves) she ever made, her dad sold his business. He moved to Hawaii and—get this—he moved there to write his first novel!

---

116   Dr. Susan Biali, "Five Steps to Finding Your Passion," *Psychology Today*, May 8, 2012.

Susan is convinced he was so upset because he wanted to do what she was doing. At the time, she was quite sure he didn't know that. But he eventually figured it out!

Fourthly, think of what you loved to do as a child. Revisit your childhood. What did you love to do? Business consultant Rob Levit suggests making a list of all the things you remember enjoying as a child.[117] Would you enjoy that activity now? For example, Frank Lloyd Wright, one of the world's greatest architects, played with wooden blocks all through childhood and perhaps well past it. Revisit some of the positive activities and events of your childhood. Levit suggests asking yourself these questions to get started: What can be translated and added into your life today? How can those past experiences shape your passion now?

Fifthly, notice when you lose track of time, or what you hate to stop doing. Notice what you love. Notice what makes you feel like a kid. Notice what you long to have more time for. It may simply be a feeling that there is nowhere else you need to be than right where you are in that moment. I always remember a seminary professor telling me that he knew he had met the woman he wanted to spend the rest of his life with when he realised that there was nowhere else he needed to be. At the time, I was still in my twenties and thought that his comments sounded very unromantic, but now, with over thirty wedding anniversaries behind me, I appreciate the truth and loveliness of what he said. So also with our calling. There is a sense that "this feels right." There is no need to be anywhere else!

---

117   Lisa Girard, "How to Find Your Passion in Five Creativity Exercises," *Entrepreneur.*

Sixth, try new things! Two dear friends have done just that! Betty learned how to swim at age fifty-five. When she and Al sold their grocery store in the small southwestern Ontario town of West Lorne, they retired to the Turks and Caicos where Al became a scuba diving instructor who took tourists on underwater journeys. Betty would listen to Al and the tourists talk endlessly about the marvels they had witnessed under the sea. Finally, she decided that she was tired of just hearing about these adventures. She wanted to share in them, too. First, she had to learn how to swim. This was a big undertaking at age fifty-five, but one she has never regretted. Soon, she was learning how to scuba dive and enjoying the splendours of deep-sea diving.

My friend and colleague, Wib, is always trying new things. Wib could very easily have fallen into the pattern of many retired clergy who provide weekly pulpit supply and part-time pastoral visitation. There's nothing wrong with that, of course, especially if one has spent time discerning one's call, not just doing this because it feels comfortable and familiar. But trying new things can be interesting and invigorating. A lifelong student, Wib is always taking new online courses, studying subjects he has never explored before. In his thirties and forties, he and a friend built an airplane and learned to fly it. Until quite recently, he loved to lead canoeing trips. In his sixties, he cycled from one end of Canada to another to raise money for the Canadian Bible Society. In addition to working on a committee to relieve homelessness in London, serving on our communications and social media committee at the church, and chairing our Healing and Wellness team at Siloam, he has taken up videography and digital painting, producing some amazing videos (some created to accompany this book) and beautiful artwork. Just the other day, he told me that he has now taken up machine knitting to help his wife make knitted prayer shawls. The important thing is not how much Wib has taken on, but that he is having fun while exploring his creative side and helping others.

So, open yourself to noticing things you might enjoy doing, and don't be afraid of getting it wrong. It's all an adventure and you are learning and growing as you go. Few things are clearer in the bible than that the God we worship loves an adventure! Through the prophet Isaiah, God proclaims: "I am about to do a new thing! Now it springs forth, do you not perceive it? I will make a way in the wilderness and rivers in the desert." (Isaiah 43:19). Look at the adventure God took with the people of Israel and, later, with the first disciples of Jesus! Happiness research shows that trying new things increases dopamine levels in the brain, contributing to sustained levels of contentment. So, try away!

Seventh, is there something you already love doing? Do you have a hobby, or something you loved doing as a child, but never considered it as a possibility? Whether it's reading comic books, collecting something, making something, creating, building, or gardening, there is probably a way you could transform it into a passion. Richard, a dedicated member of Siloam, has combined a life of community activism on behalf of one of London's needier communities with a love of wood sculpture. A retired teacher, Richard never believed that he would live to be of retirement age. His own father died young. However, together with his best friend and wife, Diana, he has taken the life God has given him and fashioned it into a retirement of great meaning and beauty. Largely because of his efforts, there is now a youth drop-in centre in northeast London, kids have a safe place to play basketball, and young families have a beautiful park in which to play as well as a safe walkway with streetlights so that they can navigate a very busy city artery to go to the local library and community centre. Together with Diana, Richard also supports Age Friendly London, furnishing local parks with benches that clearly delineate distances between each park bench so that seniors can plan their walks in comfort. Along with all this, Richard creates some of the most creative and unique wood sculptures I have ever seen.

Margaret and her sister Rhonda spent many years raising their families, volunteering for their respective church communities, and working in the professional world, where each held very responsible positions in the education field. Throughout their lives, among their many hobbies, they have enjoyed sewing and quilting. Not too long ago, they took on a new but equally creative project. They made two beautiful big church banners in memory of their parents. Truly works of art, these now hang in our Siloam sanctuary, where they are admired by members and visitors alike. They received so many compliments on these beautiful banners that they put together a most impressive wall hanging for Advent and a new banner to celebrate Siloam's 160th anniversary in 2017.

So, think of something you have always wanted to try and give it a go! Create a comic book site online. Build a community garden. Take up watercolour painting. My friend Kathy is a full-time social worker who spends her free time creating beautiful art using a variety of media. In her retirement, she plans to pursue "legacy art." As she writes, "My hope is to paint with palliative adults or children so that they can leave behind a painting for their friends or family. This would be done with one person at a time. They would choose what they wanted to paint and I would walk them through it. With children, they may paint with the help of their mom, dad, or sibling if they are unable to hold a brush. I would use acrylic paints or soft pastel. My plan would be to volunteer my services at a hospice or a family home."[118] In much the same way as a personal historian might help someone to record and write their memoirs, so Kathy will help people to create a piece of art that will become their unique legacy to the world. Kathy has loved art all her life, and she loves helping others to discover their creative gifts, so this is a natural fit for her talents. Her advice: if there's already something you love doing, you're ahead of the game.

For example, my cousin Craig has spent his whole life in the bush. A former outdoor recreation specialist at Ontario's Algonquin Park, his love of God's great outdoors began when his parents would take him and his young siblings on camping trips across North America. Every summer, they would leave the busy metropolis of Toronto behind and head for the woods. Craig would be the first to admit that he was one of the lucky ones who could turn a childhood love into a lifelong passion. In his working life, he led year-round canoe trips, engaged in rescue searches, and built and repaired trails through the forest.

Craig also became an expert on the history of the Temagami, a wilderness area that covers well over 10,000 square kilometres north of North Bay and straddles the Ontario/Quebec border. Craig has been exploring Temagami's forests, uplands, and waterways since he was a teenager. He has studied the history, language, and culture of the Anishinawbeg or Ojibway people who lived there for many generations and he has used his experience to create an important window on the land's history. His creation is called the *Historical Map of Temagami*, and it presents a unique and invaluable contribution to our understanding

---

118   Kathy Gaskin in an email to the author, July 23rd, 2017.

of the aboriginal world that existed in Canada prior to contact with the European settlers. The book was twenty-six years in the making and includes the names of 660 features—lakes, rivers, creeks, islands, and highlands—all in the language of the Anishinawbeg. It depicts traditional winter and summer travel routes and identifies hundreds of portages, along with their exact lengths. In carrying out his research, Craig estimates that he interviewed 500 native elders on Bear Island and several nearby reserves in Ontario and Quebec. He accumulated hundreds of pages of field notes and collected material on a sweeping array of things, including Anishinawbeg spiritual beliefs, conjuring methods, canoeing techniques, and places to hunt, set snares, and collect pipestones. He says, "I talked to the oldest people I could find and the younger people had trouble listening because the elders were talking about places they had never been."

His most aged informant was Phileas Lepage, who was 108 at the time of their interview and was likely born around 1868. A few days before Craig spoke to him, Lepage had had dinner with then Ontario Premier Bill Davis and Prime Minister Pierre Trudeau because, at the time, he was one of the oldest surviving veterans of World War I. Craig says that Lepage "was of such antiquity that he had seen Sir John A. Macdonald giving election speeches from the backs of trains."[119]

In the late 1980s, the Bear Island Anishinawbeg in Temagami called Craig as a witness during a land claim hearing before the Ontario Supreme Court and used his testimony to establish that their ancestors had fully utilized the land since at least the 1600s when the first French

---

119   D'Arcy Jenish, "Mapman of Temagami," *Legion Canada's Military History Magazine*, May 1, 2006.

missionaries—whom they called *way-mit-a-goosh,* or stick wavers—arrived. To this day, Craig continues to be contacted by aboriginal bands seeking similar information regarding their land claims.[120]

In his retirement, Craig runs a winter camping business, leads canoe trips, gives talks to schools and service groups, and enjoys working in his maple sugar bush. Currently, he is also writing a book on winter camping. He is blessed to have such a supportive partner in his wife Doris, who gives generously of her time to their little United Church congregation in Dorset, and who shares Craig's love of camping, at least during three seasons of the year!

Eighth, what do you spend hours reading about? Dear friends of mine read everything they could about the Camino pilgrimage and then resolved that this would be their first stop after retirement. Since then they have undertaken many walking trips throughout Europe and Canada. Or maybe your love of reading means that there is a book within you that is aching to be written. On the other hand, if, like my husband and me, you love reading Canadian, British, and Scandinavian mysteries, this does not mean that you should now embark on planning the perfect murder! It may simply mean that reading will continue to provide much pleasure in the second half of your life.

Finally, spend time cultivating your passion! Cal Newport is a computer scientist and author of four books about passion. He doesn't buy into the "follow your passion" mantra. He says, "There is no special passion

---

120   Ibid. Interestingly, it was the work of Craig's younger brother, the late Rod Macdonald, former dean and professor of law at McGill University in Montreal, that paved the way for Canada's apology to residential school survivors and was also instrumental in developing same-sex marriage legislation in Canada.

waiting for you to discover. Passion is something that is cultivated."[121] Think again about Craig's example. His passion was the result of years spent working in the bush, interviewing hundreds of First Nations elders and years of studying their ways.

Reflecting on Newport's advice, Ryan Chatterton, who counsels recent graduates on how to get a job, has developed the following equation:

$$(curiosity + engagement) \times time = passion^{122}$$

Chatterton says to start with something you are curious about (there is no "right" or "wrong" choice). Pick an interest and roll with it. It doesn't have to be something you are really excited about, just something you are curious about. Then acquire as much knowledge as you can about that subject. Read some articles or books. Watch videos about your interest.

Get Together with People Who Share Your Interests

The next thing Chatterton advises it to get together with people who share your interest. This serves two purposes.

1. First, it's easier to gather detailed knowledge from people than from static media.

2. Secondly, social engagement revolving around our interest reinforces our commitment and fuels that interest even further.[123]

---

121   Ryan Chatteron, "The Ultimate Secret to Discovering Your Passion," *The Huffington Post*, April 9, 2013.

122   . Ibid.

123   Ibid.

As he writes, there is a reason parents don't want their kids hanging out with the wrong crowd: we become like the people we hang around. "People's lives are often a direct reflection of the expectations of their peer group."[124] So, if you are interested in music, make a point of associating with other musicians, who can cheer you on and hold you accountable.

By the way, if you have never played a musical instrument before (or if it was such a long time ago that you can't remember anything about it), think about joining a band or orchestra that has been specifically designed for adults who have never played an instrument before and want to learn. Or gather some folks together, hire a music student who is keen to make some extra money, and start your own musical group!

Remember to Spend Time in Prayer and Meditation on the Scriptures

While Christians can and should take advantage of the very many real helps that exist in the secular world, our primary focus must always be on Christ and where he is calling us to serve. Consider forming an accountability circle with like-minded friends and/or people in your church who are struggling to discern where and how God is calling them to serve in the second half of life. Together, you can support one another and help to keep each other focussed on what really and truly matters: namely, your service to God.

I will always remember interviewing an elderly woman named Rena Newbery. With her husband, Ed, Rena had served the United Church of Canada in Trinidad. A recipient of the prestigious Order of Canada, she had greatly enjoyed helping to train young Trinidadians for the

---

124   Ibid.

ordained ministry, even though in her younger years, she had no idea that this was where God would be calling her to serve. One afternoon as we sat looking out her window at the beautiful autumn colours and sharing in conversation over a cup of tea, Rena said to me: "I think the question 'What do I want to become' is the wrong question for young people to ask. The question they should ask is: 'Where is God calling me into service?'" Likewise, as we age, our question should be "Where and how is God calling me to serve now?" Not "Who do I want to become?" As Rena found, this means remaining open always to the voice of God.[125]

Listening to God's call through prayer and meditation, as well as in the events around you, requires an openness to the new and often surprising ways of the Spirit. Geraldine Robertson of the Aamjiwnaang First Nation had no idea that a return in her early sixties to the reserve where she had grown up was, in fact, the Spirit calling her to live out her vocation as elder and mentor to younger generations of her band.

Geraldine was one of more than 150,000 Canadian indigenous children who were taken from their families and placed in government-funded, church-run residential schools from the 1870s through to 1996. The schools, to quote Canada's first prime minister, Sir John A. Macdonald, were built for the express purpose of "taking the Indian out of the child," and thus intended to solve what Macdonald referred to as the "Indian problem." Today, we call it cultural genocide.

Of her time at Mohawk Institute, an Anglican-run residential school in Brantford, Ont., Geraldine says: "I felt like I was living in hell." There, she was subjected to the strap nearly every day and witnessed firsthand

---

125   Personal history interviews with author, Simcoe, Ont., 2005-2006.

the sufferings of many other indigenous children who endured physical and sexual abuse. Her own sisters, who were younger and perhaps even more vulnerable than Geraldine, carried deep emotional and psychological scars that haunted them all their lives.

Later, Geraldine returned to Sarnia and made a new home for herself. But, conditioned by the school authorities never to speak of her experiences at the institute, she kept silent for sixty years. Living with her Scottish-born husband and their four children in suburban Sarnia, she never once spoke to them of the trauma she and her sisters underwent at Mohawk. Then an opportunity came for her and her husband to buy a new home on the reserve. It seemed like the thing to do now that the children were grown and away, and there was just the two of them. This would be a peaceful place in which to spend their retirement years. However, God had other plans. Geraldine had not been back long when she realised how wounded and broken many of the families on the reserve were. The young would complain to her about their parents' dysfunctional behaviour. "Moving back here, some of my cousins would tell me how their parents treated them, so I felt I had to explain what their parents went through and how it would have warped their sense of parenting."

It was then that Geraldine understood that a whole generation of First Nations children was growing up without any knowledge of the pain and suffering their parents had endured in the residential schools, separated from their own parents, and without the example of a loving and caring home life. And so, at the age of sixty, she stood before her band council and shared her own painful story of life in a residential school. Although she did not realise it at the time, the Spirit had been preparing her for sixty years for what was to become her true life's vocation as an elder to the young people of her band. She soon began to organize classes to help families understand their painful history, as well as support groups, sessions on baby wellness, and seminars on parenting skills.[126] Her work did not stop with her own community, but led her not only to speak to groups across Canada, but also to join with others in bringing a class action suit against the Government of Canada for the sufferings that she and thousands of other indigenous people had endured. Sometimes, as Geraldine discovered, "the Spirit blows where it pleases" (John 3:8, NIV), and leads us into ministries we never expected.

Discover Hidden Riches in Your Own Backyard

> *Once Jesus was asked by the Pharisees when the Kingdom of God was coming, and he answered, "The Kingdom of God is not coming with things that can be observed; nor will they say, 'Look, here it is!' or 'There it is!' For, in fact, the Kingdom of God is within you."*

– Luke 17:20-21

Harry R. Moody recounts a tale of a poor man who is discouraged by life.[127] He lives in a tumbledown cottage and scratches out a meagre living on the land surrounding it. One day, a mysterious stranger arrives at his door.

"You live in a vast mansion," the man tells him. "You just do not realise it yet."

---

126   Geraldine Robertson, interview, August 15, 2016, Aamjiwnaang First Nation.

127   Harry R. Moody and David Carroll, *The Five Stages of the Soul* (New York: Random House, 1999), 77.

The man laughs. Anyone can see his house is small and tumbling down around him. But the stranger is insistent.

Slowly, with the guidance of his new friend, the man begins to discover hidden parts of his dwelling. First, he finds one forgotten room, then another and another, until entire lavish suites are revealed. In the end, the man becomes proprietor of a thousand-room palace, a huge mansion, the same that he had once mistaken for a single dilapidated room.

Well, the story of hidden riches in one's own backyard turns up time and again in folktales and myth. The message is clear. There are hidden riches right in your own backyard!

"The Kingdom of God is within you." —*Luke 17:21*

As you reflect upon your passion and where you think God is leading you in this exciting new chapter of your life, remember these words of Jesus: "The Kingdom of God is within you." What you are looking for is hidden within yourself. Think about what makes you curious. Think about those things in which you become so engaged that you lose track of time, those things which, as Thurman wrote, "make you come alive." As spiritual writer and theologian Frederick Buechner once observed, "The place God calls you is the place where your deep gladness and the world's deep hunger meet."[128] As you go about doing the important work of discerning and planning how you will redesign the house that is your life, remember, also, those ordinary messengers who have touched your life and, through their touch, suggested another path for you.

---

128   Frederick Buechner. *Wishful Thinking: A Seeker's ABC.* (New York: Harper One, 1993), 398.

For Further Reading

Paul C. Clayton, *Called for Life. Finding Meaning in Retirement.* (Herndon, VA: The Alban Institute, 2008.)

Rena Newbery, *Sparkles on the Leaves*, as told to Sheila Macgregor, personal historian, 2006.

Moody, Harry R. and Carroll, David. *The Five Stages of the Soul.* (New York, Random House, 1999.)

For Viewing

Dewitt Jones, "For the Love of It," Training DVD and video, Star Thrower.

Re-Designing Your Life: A Practical Spirituality for the Second Half of Life, Sheila Macdonald Macgregor, Wib Dawson, videographer and editor, 2017.

Questions for Discussion

Watch Session Four of the videos that have been made to accompany this book and then discuss the following. Note: if you are leading a study group, you may not have time to discuss all the questions. Choose those that you feel will be most helpful to your group.

1. Get out your art supplies! On quality paper, use pastels or colouring pencils to draw a river to represent your life. Mark the following on your river: the headwaters or people who first introduced you to the life of faith, the places where your river drained into the lives of others, the places where your river has flowed peacefully, as well as the places where you

have encountered rocks, setbacks, and dangerous rapids. Where do you see the hand of God guiding you along the river of life?

2. Read 1 Corinthians 4:1. Canadian theologian Douglas John Hall says that this is the primary calling, not just of the clergy, but of all Christians: to be "stewards of the mysteries of God." "The quest for understanding on the part of the faithful is the work of the whole people of God." (Hall, *Bound and Free. A Theologian's Journey*, Fortress Press, 2005, p. 114.) How can the second half of life become an opportunity to live out this calling more faithfully? Why is this calling so important?

3. Read 1 Corinthians 12. Consider how you may use your own gifts and talents in service to God and your community.

4. Why does Clayton ask us to consider why it may be wrong for the Christian to identify their calling solely by way of their occupation in the first half of life? What is the difference between a job and a calling?

5. Reflecting on Jesus's passion (or work on the cross), how has your own experience of suffering shaped your life's calling or the calling of someone you know?

6. Build on the lessons of those identified in this chapter. What do you enjoy doing so much that you lose track of time? Is there something you enjoyed doing as a child that you would like to build on now in retirement? Where is God calling you to try something new for the sake of the Kingdom? Consider

joining with others who have similar interests or create an accountability group to help keep you focussed and faithful.

7. In Luke 17:21, Jesus says: "The Kingdom of God is within you." What do you think Jesus means? Is it possible that the answers you seek are already within you? How do you begin to unlock them so that you can better discern where God is calling you to serve now?

Chapter 5:
Moving in—
What to Leave Behind, What to Keep

Emptying the Closets of Life

The renovations are almost completed, and it is nearly time to move into our newly renovated house. Have we taken the time to consider our needs and carefully consider how our new home will be designed? When my husband and I began to raise our family over twenty-five years ago, closet space was always a problem. Back then, it was customary for clergy to live in a manse, a house provided by the pastoral charge and usually located next door to the church. We were always blessed with lovely manses and good manse committees, but because the houses were very old, they did not really have adequate closet space. The homes that many of my boomer friends were building during the same period, on the other hand, tended to be like small mansions and boasted large walk-in closets to accommodate our boomer appetite for more and more things. I now have such a closet and, I am ashamed to admit, it is overflowing with more stuff than I really need, which is another way to say that closets can be both a blessing and a curse.

First, closets can often be a storehouse of magical treasures. When our daughter Alexandra was just a little girl, she loved C. S. Lewis' story,

The Lion, The Witch, and the Wardrobe. She used to imagine herself as Lucy, the smallest of four young siblings who were sent off to live in a large old home in the English countryside to escape the bombings during World War II London. In the story, Lucy chances upon an interesting wardrobe, or free-standing closet, which magically also serves as a portal into a fantasy land called Narnia. Eventually, her brothers and sister also discover the magic closet and the rest of the story recounts their exciting adventures in Narnia. Alexandra loved the story so much that whenever we went shopping, she could often be found rummaging at the back of the coat racks trying to find Narnia. She used to like to play in our small closet at the manse, too, to see if it could take her to Narnia. For her, then, closets had a magical quality, filled with excitement and wonder.

Secondly, and on a sadder note, closets have not always been associated with happy places of childhood wonder. I am not just thinking of the fictional character Harry Potter who was forced by his cruel aunt and uncle to sleep in a cramped closet underneath the stairs. Of late, our news here in southwestern Ontario has been full of stories of children kept prisoner in small spaces. London, Ontario author Emma Donoghue recently won an Academy Award for the film version of her book *Room*,[129] which tells the story of a mother and her small son who, for years, are held captive in an enclosed space, not too much larger than a closet. Closets can be scary places filled with unspeakable cruelty.

There are other closets, not physical in nature but just as cruel, that have confined people over the years, forcing them to hide who they really

---

129 *Room*, directed by Lenny Abrahamson (2015), film.

are and live inauthentic lives. I am thinking here of our brothers and sisters who are gay, lesbian, trans-gendered, twin-spirited, and queer. Through its decision to ordain practising homosexuals in 1988, the United Church of Canada has played a major role in helping to release from their stifling prisons those who have been prevented because of their sexuality to live full, open lives. The pressure the church put on the Canadian government to recognize same-sex marriages in 2005 opened the closet door wider. As we continue the renovations on the house that is our life, it is important that there is space for everyone to feel welcome and accepted. This means that there are also times when we need to purge our closets of attitudes, prejudices, and behaviours that are destructive and demean members of God's family.

Here, I return to my earlier observation about the distressing nature of burgeoning boomer closets. Too many of us, myself included, find ourselves weighed down by an endless amount of stuff. There is a tendency to hoard, whether it be clothing, shoes, jewellery, books, DVDs, sports gear, or recreational vehicles. Many have commented on the need to travel lighter through the second half of life, but the idea of downsizing our property and possessions can feel daunting, to say the least. Sifting through all the piles and collections of our lives can be arduous, and we may even get lost from time to time in the process. But it is part of the important work we need to do in the second half of our lives.

Rabbi Dayle Friedman quotes an early Rabbinic text that sheds light on the issue of accumulating and divesting ourselves of all the stuff we have collected in our lives:

> Hillel used to say: "The more flesh, the more worms,
> the more possessions, the more worries, the more

wives, the more sorcery, the more servants, the more misdeeds and mistrust. [On the other hand,] the more Torah (God's word), the more life, the more study, the more wisdom, the more counsel, the more understanding, the more *tzedakah* [deeds of righteousness], the more peace.[130]

The urge to have more brings only increased worry and unhappiness. Unburdening ourselves from years of piled-up papers, books, and the endless amount of stuff we collect can help us to move from acquiring things or people, to freeing us to share our wisdom with others. In the letting go of all this stuff, moreover, there is the possibility that life will be enriched in ways we could never have imagined. As Friedman writes, "You're not just giving up, you're *getting*."[131] You don't have to spend as much time cleaning, dusting, and worrying about your stuff. Plus, the open spaces will give you room to breathe!

The closet has other lessons to teach us, as I discovered years ago, as I was getting ready to head off on a Rotary Fellowship to St. Andrews, Scotland. Before I left, I decided that it was time to purge my closet. I knew it could be a few years before I would be home again, and since my parents did not have a lot of storage space in their house, it did not seem fair for me to hold that closet hostage while I was away. More importantly, I knew that there were a lot of clothes that I would likely never wear again, and I thought that someone else could get some enjoyment from them. As I began to load all my old belongings into

---

130   Rabbi Dayle A. Friedman, *Jewish Wisdom for Growing Older. Finding Your Grit & Grace Beyond Midlife.* (Woodstock, VT: For People of All Faiths, All Backgrounds, Jewish Lights Publishing, 2015), 101.

131   Ibid., 102.

bags to take to the Goodwill, my mother offered, helpfully, "Oh, don't worry about those things now. I will take them to the Goodwill for you." Some years later, I happened to be home staying in my former bedroom. I opened the closet door and, lo and behold, there were all my old clothes. They had never made it to the Goodwill. When I asked my mother about them, she said that she had decided to save them. Clothing, she insisted, always comes back in style and she thought I would want to wear these castoffs again. What my mother did not understand, however, is that, while fashions do often come back in style, figures seldom remain the same. Certainly, after four ten-pound babies, there was no chance my figure would ever fit into those clothes again, no matter how stylish they were. At the time, I was secretly upset with my mother for not taking the clothes to the Goodwill as she had promised. Someone else could have enjoyed them during the years I had been away. However, with several more years of hindsight, and our eldest son Lachlan now teaching across the ocean in Marrakech, I now understand that this was not simply about the frugal values of a Depression-era mother. At least, that was not the only reason she had saved the clothes. It was about hanging onto her only daughter, the close friendship we shared, and the memories of all the fun we had in buying those clothes, since we nearly always shopped together. Most of all, I suspect that it was also about her understanding of herself as my mother. Maybe if she hung onto these clothes, I would one day come back to live in my hometown and life would be the same again.

Friedman would have understood what was going on that summer, as my mother contemplated her daughter leaving the nest. She has spent the past thirty years ministering to and learning from older adults. Her most recent book is *Jewish Wisdom for Growing Older: Finding Your*

Grit and Grace Beyond Midlife. There, she writes, "Relinquishing things that hold memories makes us feel at risk of losing our connection to the past, particularly to people and relationships that are gone."[132] The empty closet was a painful reminder to my mother that her nest had just got smaller.

Today, as I write this, it is the twentieth anniversary of my mother's death. How well I recall my own feelings of sadness and loss as I sorted through her closet after she died. For my father, it was even tougher. Every morning, he would open his dresser drawer and just gaze at the shirts my mother had washed, ironed, and neatly folded and placed there. Sometimes he would pick one of the shirts up and caress it in his hands, but he never wore any of the shirts again. He just wanted to look at them and touch them, knowing that the last hands that had placed them there were my mother's. Probably the least fashion-conscious person I have ever known, Dad could not have cared less about the shirts. It was the connection to my mother that they provided that he could not bear to lose.

Letting Go

Franciscan priest Richard Rohr says that the acquisition of material things is a "first-half-of-life" preoccupation.[133] There is nothing wrong with material goods in and of themselves. Such things fit together with other first-half-of-life endeavours like getting an education, buying a car, building a career, and establishing a home, an identity, family, friends, and so on. One needs to navigate these important tasks with some degree of success to make a smooth transition to the second

---

132 Ibid., 101.

133 Richard Rohr, *Falling Upward: A Spirituality for the Two Halves of Life.* (San Francisco: Jossey-Bass, 2011), viii.

half of life. The problem, Rohr says, is that we are a "'first-half-of-life culture,' largely concerned about surviving successfully."[134]

Rohr notes that, in contrast to the agenda of the first half of life, the second half of life is about spiritual maturity and the art of learning to "let go." He says, "All great spirituality teaches about letting go of what you don't need and who you are not. Then, when you can get little enough and naked enough and poor enough, you'll find that the little place where you really are is ironically more than enough and is all that you need. At that place, you will have nothing to prove to anybody and nothing to protect."[135] It may seem ironic that, at the same time the blessings of modern medicine provide many of us with a whole extra room at the centre of our lives, we need to clear away much of the debris and clutter of the first half of life in order to fully inhabit this new space. The atrium at the centre of our life is indeed only possible to the extent that we let go of much of what we depended on in the first half of life.

Elsewhere, Rohr describes how "letting go" is the basis of our freedom in Christ:

> Authentic spirituality is always on some level or in some way about letting go. Jesus said, "the truth will set you free" (John 8:32). Once we see truly what is trapping us and keeping us from freedom we should see the need to let it go. But in a consumer society, most of us have had no training in that direction. Rather, more is supposed to be better. True liberation is letting go of our false self, letting go of our cultural biases,

---

134   Ibid., viii–xv, 2.

135   Richard Rohr, *Healing Our Violence Through the Journey of Centering Prayer* (Albuquerque, NM: Centre for Action and Contemplation, 2013), CD.

and letting go of our fear of loss and death. Freedom is letting go of wanting more and better things, and it is letting go of our need to control and manipulate God and others. It is even letting go of our need to know and our need to be right—which we only discover with maturity. We become free as we let go of our three primary energy centers: our need for power and control, our need for safety and security, and our need for affection and esteem.[136]

Like Mary Magdalene as she meets the resurrected Jesus in the garden, the message we hear in the second half of life is: "Do not hold onto me." (John 20:17) On a purely practical level, this means relaxing our grip on all the material possessions and achievements that have defined us to date. Secondly, and more importantly, it means that we must not cling to preconceived notions of God or how life should be. In this stage, we finally realise that we cannot control our lives and we certainly cannot control God. Letting go means becoming vulnerable to the Spirit and opening ourselves up to where God is calling us.

Benedictine nun Joan Chittister observes that, instead of being preoccupied with material things, this period of the spirit is for shaping the soul. As she writes, "Every major tradition knows as one of its core experiences a period of major divestment, of total renunciation of that which shaped a person before he or she began the great spiritual quest."[137] Chittister writes that this is a time for considering the

---

136   Adapted from Richard Rohr, *The Art of Letting Go: Living the Wisdom of Saint Francis* (Sounds True), CD.

137   Joan Chittister. *The Gift of Years: Growing Older Gracefully* (New York: Blue Bridge, 2008), 91.

meaning of life and death and "for stripping ourselves of whatever we have accrued until this time in order to give ourselves wholly to the birthing of the person within."[138] In other words, for something new to be born, we need to practise the art of "letting go," or what the biblical writers refer to as the dying unto self.

The theme of dying unto self is part of the focus of the beautiful book about conscious elderhood written by Anne Beattie-Stokes. As we saw earlier, Beattie-Stokes discovered that her role as an elder is to create for others a safe place in which to die. In her training to become a conscious elder herself, she learned that her own "ministry is to help people die in every stage of life—to faith that is too small, to self-images that are too small, to views of the world that are too small, to the stage of life that is ending, and, finally, to life itself."[139] These are the toughest kinds of "letting go" that any of us will ever do, but they are also necessary if we are to experience spiritual renewal.

In her guide to the midlife spirit, former United Church of Canada moderator Mardi Tindal says that "it was amazing how often the theme of "letting go" came up in [her] conversations with other midlifers—letting go of burdensome possessions, ambitions, expectations of the exuberance of youth; of the presence of loved ones."[140] In her own life, Tindal says that this has meant having to give up the ability to work from dawn until midnight, as well as being forced to give up the presence of parents and friends who have died. As we get ready to move into our newly renovated house, there are some closets that need to be

---

138   Ibid.

139   Beattie-Stokes, *A Heart of Wisdom*, 7, 20–21, 23.

140   Mardi Tindal, *Soul Maps: A Guide to the Mid-Life Spirit* (Toronto: United Church Publishing House, 2000), 29.

emptied of their contents, or at least streamlined. There are also certain pieces of furniture that just won't fit. There are pictures and ornaments and other knickknacks that suited the old home, but which now seem out of place. This is a time for simplifying our living space and for letting go of all the things that only create clutter and confusion.

For some of us, our closet purge will be quite radical, and we will need to leave nearly everything behind. Recall the story of Naomi in the Old Testament. Economic refugees, she and her husband and two sons were forced to flee their home in Israel for the land of Moab. There, her sons married Moabite women. There, also, her husband died and, after him, both of Naomi's sons died as well, leaving no children behind, only their wives. One daughter-in-law, Ruth, chose to stay with Naomi and journey with her mother-in-law to Israel. The *Book of Ruth* is the beautiful story of their love and faithfulness to each other. Their story begins, however, with these brief but telling words: Naomi "went forth out of the place where she was" (Ruth 1:7 KJV). The scriptures say nothing about Naomi packing up her bags and loading her luggage on the back of the camel. She doesn't line her pockets with any souvenirs to remind her of her time in Moab. She just gets up and leaves it all behind. Some of us in midlife will need to do the same.

That said, this does not mean for others of us that there won't be some material possessions that we will want to carry with us into the redeveloped space that is our life. My father had a comfortable but rather dowdy old chair where he would sit every day to read and meditate. My mother hated that chair with a passion and would have loved to have replaced it with something new and stylish, but Dad would not hear of it. If you ever watched the popular sitcom *Frasier,* you will know how insistent Martin was that he be allowed to keep his tattered, worn, but much-loved recliner, even though it did not fit with his son Frasier's classy, uptown decor. The point is clear. Whatever assists us to do the work we need to do in this new phase of our lives should be kept. Anything that gets in the way of our life task should be discarded. Sometimes, that means keeping the tattered old chair and losing the need for keeping up appearances.

In my own life, I think that one of the things I need to leave behind in the second half is something I have struggled with my whole life long: namely, the belief that I can do it all. When I entered theological college in the late seventies, women were just beginning to flood the previously male-dominated seminary halls (even though the first time a woman was ordained in the United Church of Canada occurred some forty years earlier, when Lydia Gruchy was ordained in 1936). Few Canadians realise that for nearly thirty years thereafter, only single women could be ordained to the ministry of Word and Sacraments. I still remember the older female colleague who called on me one day to congratulate me on my recent ordination and to see my new baby. My heart broke as she told me that when she was ordained back in the mid-1950s, she had to choose between getting married and having a family or going into full-time ordained ministry. My generation of women, on the other hand, had been given choices that had never been available to her. That said, because the doors now seemed to open wide to my sisters in ministry and me, many of us believed we could do it all and have it all—a full-time ministry in the church *and* a family—and we nearly killed ourselves in the process! Moreover, because we were still trying to prove that we could minister just as effectively as our male counterparts, we often burnt the candle at both ends. To this day, I profoundly regret a decision I made to leave my two-year-old daughter and her three-week-old baby brother to take part in a three-day meeting several hours from where we lived. While I had a wonderfully supportive husband and a dear friend who loved the children as her own, my place in those early days should have been at home enjoying this precious time with my little ones. I would like to say that I learned my lesson by the time my two younger sons were born, but that would not be true. I was still trying to keep up with the guys. The good news is that in the last few years I have witnessed real changes taking place in the lives of my younger colleagues, male and female, who have better personal boundaries when it comes to protecting their family time. My former colleague in ministry at Siloam, Rev. Isaac Mundy, is a fine example of a young and uniquely gifted minister who serves the church faithfully, but not at the expense of his wife and children. His call to the ministry of Word and Sacraments does not undermine or diminish his call to be a husband and father. That's progress. It's also good news for his congregation because churches are healthier when their clergy have a healthy home life, too.

Whether we have served in the church or spent our working years in business, industry, education, health care, or raising a family—and whether we are male, female, or transgendered—part of the task for this new stage will be to simplify our life and reduce the amount of busy work we do. The home we build will need to have space—not for yet one more project, but rather for reflection and discernment.

It goes without saying that, along with all the above, there is another kind of "letting go" we must do in this period of our lives. As Tindal says, this "may be the hardest thing to let go of,"[141] namely, the roles we have come to assume in life:

> The parts we play have been developed over many
> years and with great investment and practice to get

---

141   Ibid.

them right. No one is standing in the wings with a new script to replace the old. Once we let go, as we must, we must start from scratch, often feeling empty and disoriented.[142]

The writer of *First Peter* reminds us that, as disciples of Jesus, we have an identity that transcends all the various parts and roles we have played in life: "you are a chosen people, a royal priesthood, a holy nation . . ." (1 Peter 2:9). Tragically, our lives have been bombarded by advertisements, as well as by well-meaning family and friends, that tell us that our identity comes from the jobs or positions we hold, the number of degrees that bedeck our walls, or the size of our bank account and the model of car we drive. The result is that we have lost sight of our true identity as the children of God. Sometimes. I feel we in the church are plagued by Korsakov's Syndrome. We suffer severe memory loss—not from alcohol abuse, but, rather, from cultural abuse, which leads us to confabulate stories about who we are in much the same way that sufferers of Korsakov's Syndrome make up stories to fill in the gaps in their memory. The result is just as deadly, as we buy into false identities that have nothing to do with our God-given identity as God's precious children.

Perhaps by pruning our over-programmed and over-busy schedules, we can begin to carve out some space to recover our God-given identity and for discerning what is truly important now. What is this time in our lives meant for? As Friedman writes, "Perhaps this time of life is an opportunity for discovering new ways to inhabit time. If we have been busy, busy, busy all the time, we might experiment with designating time to simply *be*."[143]

---

142   Ibid., p. 31.

143   Friedman, *Jewish Wisdom for Growing Older*, 107.

Her words are echoed by Canadian researcher Jane Kuepfer, who says: "I think Boomers have learned to treat busyness as a virtue, which has undermined them at times in life. Now I see as Boomers retire, many are getting a different perspective on time.... There's a reclaiming of spaciousness of time that I think has the potential to happen for Boomers, because they're not necessarily as busy as they think they are.... And there are some great ways to use time that aren't about being busy."[144] This period will be a good opportunity for us to discern not only what we need to leave behind, but also what we want to keep as we move into the house that will become our home in the second half of life.

Keepers of Meaning

In the thirteenth chapter of *Exodus* and the nineteenth verse is found this brief, seemingly insignificant statement: "And Moses took the bones of Joseph with him . . ."

The people of Israel had lived under the whip and lash of the Egyptian slave masters for 400 years. Then, from among the Hebrews, God raised up Moses to lead them from their bondage, to organize them into a nation, and to take them to the freedom of the Promised Land. After Moses attempted to negotiate their release with the pharaoh, aided by ten plagues, the time of their departure finally came. Moses commanded the slaves to pack quickly and secretly, and when the hour approached, to make haste to leave. The bible indicates that, within hours, nearly a million Israelites moved out of Egypt: "And Moses took with him the bones of Joseph...." (Exodus 13:19)

---

144   Interview with Jane Kuepfer, Thursday, July 27th, 2017.

Now, why drag along the bones of a patriarch who had been dead for two centuries? Well, remember that Joseph was the spoiled little Jewish boy who was sold by his jealous brothers in Palestine to Egyptian tradesmen who, in turn, took him to Memphis. With his ability and talent, Joseph, upon maturity, became a statesman, the prime minister, no less, of Egypt. In this favoured position, led by his faith in God, he brought his Jewish kinsmen and women to Egypt when a famine threatened their existence. Joseph excelled in faith, in moral practice, in wisdom, and in leadership. The people had to take his bones with them on their forty-year journey, so they would not forget his righteousness, his leadership, his faith, and his wisdom. So "Moses took with him the bones of Joseph…" By this recall, they would know they were a keeper of destiny.

Back in Chapter One, I referred to the psychiatrist George Vaillant, who describes those entering the second half of life as the "keepers of meaning." They are the ones who dispense wisdom and experience to the next generation. The "keepers of meaning," Vaillant maintains, are not simply concerned with the care of individuals, but with preserving the culture's traditions. If we use the biblical language of the *Book of Exodus*, they are the ones who have been charged with the task of carrying the bones of Joseph with them.

Bridges once talked about attending a conference where many businesses and organizations had booths set up in the entranceway or narthex of the convention hall. These businesses were advertising their work. A company that helped other organizations relocate their personnel to and from overseas assignments had a booth there advertising its services. At the booth, it gave away as advertising little packets of stickers that a person in transit could use to communicate with movers.[145] There were four labels in the packet. They read as follows:

> **AIR:** This was to be used for important things that you would need at the new location immediately.
>
> **SEA:** This was for things that you wanted to take along, but that were not so important as to require fast transit.
>
> **STORAGE:** This sticker was to be used with things that you didn't want to discard, but that you also knew you really didn't want to use just now.
>
> **THIS STAYS:** This was to be put on things that you realised that it was time to get rid of and leave behind.

It is time to consider how we might use these stickers in our lives as we move—not from one geographical region to another, but into this new phase of our lives. We are mostly interested in the first two stickers. We have already considered some of the things we need to leave behind. Now that the renovations to our house are nearly completed, what do we want to keep from our old house? What do we want to keep from the past? What are our non-negotiables? What do we want to bring into our newly renovated space? What are the bones we want to carry with us?

What from the old life do we want to preserve?

To figure this out, we're going to look first at what motivates us—or what has motivated us in the past.

---

145   Bridges, *The Way of Transition*, 72.

Psychologist David McClelland says he believes that "a person's motivation and effectiveness can be increased through an environment [that] provides them with their ideal mix of each of the three needs"—the needs for affiliation, power, and achievement. These needs can be described simply:[146]

> **The Need for Affiliation:** The need for friendly interactions, popularity, and a deep sense of community makes people with this need good team players.

> **The Need for Power:** Some people feel a need for personal power over others—not a desirable quality. Others desire institutional power, seeking to direct the efforts of the team—a positive contribution to the community.

> **The Need for Achievement:** Some need to excel and succeed; they enjoy working on their own and don't need praise. Their achievement is all the reward they need.

McClelland used his research to improve leadership. But, as Clayton notes, it can also be used to enhance our retirement or how we navigate the second half of life.[147] If we understand our need for affiliation, power, or achievement, we can shape our retirement or second half of life to meet that need. The volunteer assignments, the groups we join, and the hobbies we develop will be different for each motivating

---

146 Clayton, *Called for Life,* 52-53. David McClelland, *Human Motivation Theory,* www.learnmanagement2.com/DavidMcClelland.htm.

147 Ibid.

inclination. In planning ahead, we need to recognize what has motivated us in the past.

Create a Life, Not a Lifestyle

As a baby boomer, I am part of the most-targeted market that has ever existed. Marketers have carefully researched the consumer values of boomers, which are different from previous generations. They are now creating products and pitches that appeal to boomer values. Basically, they want to sell my cohorts and me a lifestyle. They want us to value consuming the right investments, the right insurance, the right real estate, the right travel, the right retail goods, and the right anti-aging products. Instead of discovering our identity, they want to sell us an identity, or at least they want us to identify ourselves as a consumer. So, if we buy all the right stuff, we'll have the right lifestyle. We'll have the "good life." The challenge that lies before us and all who enter the second half of life is this: Do we want to be sold a *lifestyle* dreamed up by an advertising agency? Or do we want to design a *life* based on our own values?

Remember the story of Adam and Eve and the snake in the Garden of Eden? Are you going to create your own life or are you going to leave it to the snake or the advertising agencies that want to sell you a lifestyle but who cannot give you a life?

Since you are reading this book, I assume that you want to design a life, not purchase a lifestyle. So I invite you to think again about those times in your life when you have felt most excited or engaged by what you were doing, when, in Thurman's words, you felt most alive.

Martin Seligman and Happiness

For a long time now, we have spent a lot of time and billions of dollars to create a mountain of detailed knowledge about the 1,001 ways that people become unhappy. This is important information because there are many people who need the help that good research into this discipline can provide.

To balance out all this knowledge about unhappiness, a new discipline called positive psychology emerged around the turn of the new millennium. This is not just a variation on "positive thinking." The inquiry into positive psychology was championed by the renowned research psychologist Martin Seligman and others. Thanks to the findings of this new discipline, we now know about approaches for increasing our "psychological well-being." Personally, I think that this is something that people of faith have known about for centuries—but more about this later.

Seligman suggests that there are, essentially, three approaches to happiness; that is, three basic ways to be happy. There are, of course, an unlimited number of specific ways to be happy, but the approaches come down to three basic ones: pleasure, engagement, and meaning.[148]

Pleasure or Enjoyment:

The kinds of things that may bring us pleasure are things like the following:

---

148   John E. Nelson and Richard N. Bolles, *What Colour is Your Parachute? For Retirement.* Second Edition. (Berkeley: Ten Speed Press, 2013), Chapter 9. Martin E. P. Seligman, *Flourish: A Visionary New Understanding of Happiness and Well-Being,* (New York: Free Press, 2011), Chapter 1. *Authentic Happiness: Using the New Positive Psychology to Realise Your Potential for Lasting Fulfillment.* (New York, NY: Free Press, 2002).

- an afternoon at a ball game;

  lunch with a friend;

  an entertaining movie or play;

  a game of golf or tennis or swimming at the beach;

  a romantic dinner with a spouse or BBQ with friends or extended family;

  a nice holiday or a weekend at the cottage.

Seligman would argue that pleasure brings a burst of positive emotions that come and go quickly. The pleasure doesn't usually last much longer than the events themselves, and we often need to go back and do these things again and again, to get more happiness. There is nothing wrong with this. We all need to do things that bring us pleasure. But we need to understand that these things, in and of themselves, do not bring lasting happiness or fulfilment.

Engagement or Involvement

Positive psychology researcher Mihaly Csikszentmihalyi[149] uses another word for this kind of happiness, an experience you can almost feel. He calls it "flow." Flow happens when your abilities are well matched to some challenging task. You get so deep into the activity, whatever it is, that you lose all track of time. You may feel like it's been only a few minutes, but it's been much longer. Either way, when you're that engaged, you lose yourself

---

149   Nelson & Bolles. *What Colour is Your Parachute? For Retirement,* 2nd ed., Chapter 9, p. 192.

in what you are doing. You may not even be aware that it makes you happy *while* you are doing it, but, *afterward,* you say, "That was great!"

Engagement involves challenge, and it demands something from you, so it's not as simple as pleasure. It can't be purchased or consumed in the way that pleasure can be. When you use this approach, it can stick with you longer than pleasure does. Over time, it can build up into a lasting satisfaction with life.

Remember: flow is about enjoyable effort. It isn't even remotely like the laid-back, whatever attitude of "go with the flow." No, this second level is more like "make the flow."

Example: Let's say you're interested in baseball. You could choose to be a spectator at a baseball game, or you could choose to be a player on a team. The low level of skill needed to be a spectator would produce a pleasant experience, but the higher level of skill needed to be a player would produce an engaging experience.

Meaning

The way you get this kind of happiness is to use your abilities in the service of something larger than yourself. Like engagement, this approach requires something from you, too. Note that meaning doesn't come from just believing in something larger than yourself; it comes from being in service to that something.

What's larger than yourself? God, your religious faith, your family, the environment, your community, your political party, a safer neighbour-hood, the sick, the needy, our educational and health-care systems. It may not be service to something larger than yourself but to something beyond yourself: a neighbour who needs help with chores, a child who needs help with school, a cleaner and litter-free walking path, or more green space or age-friendly parks that young and old can both enjoy.

We can't buy or consume meaning, just as we cannot buy or consume engagement. And contributing your money to something you believe in doesn't provide the same sense of meaning or happiness that working for it provides.[150]

This is very biblical. Remember, Jesus said: "For those who want to save their life will lose it, and those who lose their life for my sake will find it." (Matthew 16:25). There is real truth in that. As we saw in an earlier chapter, this was Albert Schweitzer's secret to true happiness, too.

Your Strengths

Now that you have a better idea of where your passion lies—or what really engages you and gives you meaning—consider the strengths on which you can build. This next step is important. Identifying and building on our strengths is going to be a major factor in our successful transition to the second half of life.

There are lots of exercises you can do to determine your strengths. Some require an hour or several hours of your time to complete. The following is a quick way to learn more about your gifts and strengths, developed by Cambridge-educated Marcus Buckingham.[151]

On a piece of paper and in point form, describe a task or activity that you have done about which you can say:

Ibid.

ela Walsh, "Marcus Buckingham: Your Strengths & What Gives You ·" *Potential Within: Reflective Writing through Yoga. Balancing Effort and ·d off the Mat* (blog), July 12, 2008.

1. You are really good at this;

2. When thinking about the task, you are *excited*—you anticipate the activity;

3. When doing the task, you find it easy to concentrate and get
   absorbed in the activity, even losing track of time;

4. Once the task is completed, you have more energy
   than before.

Share your findings with a friend whom you really trust. Ask for their
honest feedback, and then do the same for them!

Grandparents Are Important: What Kind of Legacy Do You Want to Leave?

There is no question that many men and women derive great meaning
from sharing life with their grandchildren or great-nieces and great-
nephews. Indeed, in nearly all the interviews I conducted with those in
life's second half, this theme has emerged again and again.

One of the pioneers in ministry to those in the second half of life is
Amy Hansen. Hansen has written extensively on the subject. I love
the story she tells about a time she was speaking with a very dedicated
retired gentleman. She asked him how it happened that he devoted so
much of his time to serving his church and community. Here's what
he said:

"When my granddaughter was a little girl, I used to sing a song to her
that went like this:

'One, two, three, four, five, six, seven,
All good girls go to heaven.
When they get there, they will say,
We love Jesus every day.'

"One day, I overheard her singing the song in another room.
She sang:

'One, two, three, four, five, six, seven,
All good grandpas go to heaven.
When they get there, they will say,
'GOLF, GOLF, GOLF, GOLF, every day!
"WE LOVE JESUS EVERY DAY.'"

At this point, Amy says that she cracked up laughing, but he looked her straight in the eyes with a serious look on his face and said, "Amy, in that moment, I saw myself through the eyes of my granddaughter. She saw what my passion was, and this was not the legacy I wanted to leave."[152]

Now, there was nothing wrong with this man's desire to play golf. In fact, it should, indeed, find a place in his social portfolio, since it can bring him exercise, quality time with friends and acquaintances, and fun. It is a pleasure that he should keep on his schedule. But as he himself came to understand, it's a hobby that needs to be balanced with those things that engage one's soul and which bring true meaning.

Such things include spending time with your grandchildren or great-nieces and nephews. Recent studies have shown, for example, that children benefit greatly from time spent with grandparents. Indeed,

---

152 Amy Hanson, *Baby Boomers and Beyond: Tapping the Ministry Talents and Passions of Adults Over 50,* (San Francisco: Jossey-Bass, 2010), 185, Loc. 3037.

author Penelope Farmer even goes so far as to assert that "What everyone needs in the (new) millennium is access to the internet and a grandmother."[153]

You see, one thing we do know is that grandparents have played a key role in the lives of their grandchildren. Anthropologists Sarah Blaffer Hrdy and Kristen Hawkes argue that grandmothers especially have been important to human evolution and development. Hawkes writes: "Grandmothering was the initial step toward making us who we are."[154] In the hunter-gatherer age, grandmothers could help to collect food and feed children before they were able to feed themselves. This enabled a mother to have more children, especially if she already had a young toddler. Indeed, without the assistance from grandmothers, the odds of that young toddler surviving would be much lower because human children are not able to feed themselves immediately after they have been weaned.[155] Grandmothers could and did literally often mean the difference between life and death for these youngsters!"[156]

While we don't know a lot about grandparents in the bible, we do have a few examples of men and women who blessed the lives of their grandchildren. Those today who have adopted their grandchildren will see a scriptural precedent in the actions of Jacob, who both

---

153   Sarah Blaffer Hrdy, *Mothers and Others. The Evolutionary Origins of Mutual Understanding.* (Cambridge, M.A., Bellknap Press, 2009), chapter 8, Loc. 4142 or 9574.

154   Sarah Blaffer Hrdy, Ibid., chapter 8.

155   Joseph Stromberg, "New Evidence That Grandmothers Were Crucial for Human Evolution," smithsonian.com, October 23, 2012.

156   Sadly, this is still the case in many countries in Africa where the AIDS epidemic has left many children without mothers and fathers and where grandparents have had to step in to raise their grandchildren.

blessed and adopted two of his grandsons by sons Joseph, Ephraim, and Manasseh. Then there's Hannah, mother of the famous prophet Samuel. While Hannah's grandsons did not turn out to be model leaders, Hannah herself was a faithful and prayerful servant of God. Naomi's faithfulness and courage are legendary. We can imagine that she was a good grandmother to Obed, who fathered Jesse, who later fathered King David. In the New Testament, we also have the fine example of Lois, who was very influential in the life of her grandson, the pastor and evangelist, Timothy.

Today's grandmothers—and grandfathers, too—may still help with meals from time to time, but (in the West, at least) their refusal or inability to assist does not mean their grandchildren will suffer from starvation. But the practical and emotional support they give to young families is very real. Grandparents provide much-needed babysitting support. They provide transportation, ferrying grandkids to school, to hockey and ballgames, to dance and piano lessons, and to a host of other activities, sometimes providing important financial support for these programs. In our church at Siloam, it is frequently the grandparents or great-aunts who bring the children to worship and Sunday School, or to Vacation Bible School in the summertime. As Will Randolph reminded us, grandparents often play a key role in the spiritual development of the children in our midst.

While there is still much more research that needs to be done, current studies show that grandparents are now playing an increasing role in their grandchildren's lives. University of Oxford professor Ann Buchannan has demonstrated in her work, for example, that "a high level of grandparental involvement increases the well-being of children."[157] Those children who have greater interaction with their grandparents have been shown to suffer from fewer emotional and behavioural problems. This is especially true of adolescents whose parents have undergone a divorce or separation. Buchanan's research also highlights the vital role that grandfathers play in children's lives. As she notes, "whereas grandmothers are more involved in nurturing, grandfathers get involved in activities and mentoring." [158]

You don't need to be the best grandparent ever. Just being there for your grandchildren is what counts. Hugs and cuddles, reading to them, engaging them in conversation, going for walks together, playing games, watching their baseball and hockey games, and providing a shoulder to cry on, all make a positive difference in the lives of grandchildren, especially if these activities are carried out in real time, face to face.[159]

But that's not all. Such activities also contribute to greater happiness and well-being for the grandparents. Interestingly, Buchanan's studies show that grandparents who are more involved in their grandchildren's lives are likelier to have better physical and emotional health themselves. So the benefits are two-way.

Family educator Susan McKane says that "the most wonderful thing about being a grandparent is seeing your grandchild's face light up

---

157   Ann Buchanan and Julia Griggs, "My Second Mum and Dad. The Involvement of Grandparents in Teenage Grandchildren" in *Grandparents Plus*, Report/ August 2009.

158   Ibid.

159   Susan Pinker, *The Village Effect. How Face-to-Face Contact Can Make Us Healthier and Happier.* (Toronto, Vintage Canada, 2015), pp. 139, 345.

when you walk into the room."[160] It is pure joy. At a recent grandparenting workshop that Susan led at my church, she told of her friend, a widow, who called to say she had fallen in love. When asked who the exciting new man in her life was, her friend replied that it was her three-month-old grandson!

Such feelings are not unusual. Ric, a retired school principal, says that becoming a grandfather is one of the best things that has ever happened to him. When he is talking about his grandchildren, his face bursts into the biggest smile you have ever seen, and he beams proudly. He says, "There's nothing like it! It's wonderful!" His wife, Susan, agrees wholeheartedly. A close, happy couple, they say that grandparenting has brought them more joy than they could ever have imagined. I know several great-aunts and great-uncles who play a similar role in the lives of their great-nieces and -nephews who would concur. The benefits are mutual. Both children and the older adults in their lives are blessed by these relationships and are likely healthier physically and emotionally because of them.

McKane notes another important benefit that comes with grandparenting. She says that "becoming a grandparent is like being given a second chance." She quotes her husband, Rev. Dr. David McKane, who is fond of saying that "you get to make up for all the mistakes you made as parents." Moreover, "you don't need to take over the parents' role of judge or disciplinarian."[161] You just get to enjoy!

As grandparents spend time with their grandchildren, they create memories that will be treasured long after the grandchildren have

---

160   Interview with Susan McKane, Wednesday, July 5th, 2017.
161   Ibid.

grown to adulthood and perhaps have grandchildren of their own. Interestingly, Ric says that until he became a grandparent, he found himself constantly looking back, wondering whether his parents would approve of what he was doing or whether they would be pleased with the family and career he had built. Now that he has young grandchildren of his own, he finds himself looking to the future, asking what kind of legacy he can create for the next generation.

Another important way that grandparents can share a legacy with their grandchildren is through the writing of an ethical will.

Creating an Ethical Will [162] *or Legacy Letter*

> *As the Father has loved me, so I have loved you; abide in my love.* [10] *If you keep my commandments, you will abide in my love, just as I have kept my Father's commandments and abide in his love.* [11] *I have said these things to you so that my joy may be in you, and that your joy may be complete.*
>
> [12] *"This is my commandment, that you love one another as I have loved you." (John 15:9–12)*

What is an ethical will? It is probably the best way I know to help people figure out what is really important to them in this journey called life and what they would like to share with the next generation. It is a good place to consider how we become "keepers of meaning" and how we live out of our generativity.

---

162   Barry K. Baines, *Ethical Wills: Putting Your Values on Paper* (Boston: Da Capo Press, 2002).

Some years ago, I took a course in Minneapolis with Dr. Barry Baines, in which he outlined what he means by ethical will. Baines spent his medical career dealing with patients who were palliative. Every week, he and his medical team, which consisted of oncologists and other specialists, nurses, social workers, and counsellors would meet to discuss the condition of their patients. Together, they worked to provide the best possible care to their terminally ill patients and to make their time in the palliative wing of the hospital as comfortable and as pain-free as was medically possible.

One day, one of the team members presented the case of a man who was deeply depressed. While they had managed to control the man's physical pain and keep him relatively comfortable, he had slipped into a dark state of depression. He was filled with guilt and remorse over the kind of legacy he was leaving his family. What could they do to help him?

It was then that Baines was reminded of a tradition from his own Jewish faith: the practice of writing a kind of farewell letter to one's family and friends. Baines suggested that the counsellor work with the man and help him to write a letter to his loved ones, telling them how much he loved them, recounting some of his accomplishments in life, things he regretted and for which he offered an apology, and the good things he wished for his family in the future, after he was gone.

An extraordinary thing happened. The man perked right up. His spirits lifted and gradually he emerged from out of the pit of his sadness. He started to feel better about his life, what he had achieved, and became hopeful for his family's future, too. Baines says that the man underwent an amazing transformation of the spirit.

Thus, the modern ethical will was born. Succinctly put, an ethical will is a way to share your values, blessings, life's lessons, hopes and dreams for the future, love, and forgiveness with your family, friends, and community. Sometimes called a legacy letter, it can be written and shared at any point in life, not just near the end. In fact, it is often best if you share it with your loved ones long before you die. While not a legal document, it can help you to decide what is truly important in your life and what kind of legacy you want to leave, and so be an important first step in preparing a living will and your last will and testament, which are legal wills.

Some people write their ethical will when a baby is born, or a child goes off to university or gets married. Sometimes, they write it on the occasion of a grandchild's birth. They may also update it at various times in their life, especially when there is a significant milestone. Sometimes a codicil may be added at the time of a divorce, serious illness, or death.

As you will have guessed, ethical wills are not new. The Hebrew bible first described ethical wills 3,000 years ago (Genesis 49). References to this tradition are also found in the Christian bible (John 14–18, particularly John 15, above) and in other cultures. Initially, ethical wills were transmitted orally. Over time, they evolved into written documents. Today, ethical wills are being written by people at turning points in their lives: when they're facing challenging life situations and at transitional life stages. Ethical wills may be one of the most cherished and meaningful gifts you can leave to your family and community. What's more, you don't have to have a lot of money to share this kind of legacy. Ethical wills are about values, not valuables. They are about things of the spirit, and everyone can leave a spiritual legacy.

Perhaps the best reason for people to consider writing an ethical will is that it is a good exercise for determining what really and truly and ultimately matters to us and how we want to live out our values and dreams as we move into this new phase of life. What are the things we want to let go of as we move into our newly renovated house? My guess is that we want to leave behind the stress of the day-to-day job, the tight schedules, petty politics, and any jealousies, rivalries, or disappointments we may have encountered in our working career. On the other hand, we will likely want to keep some of the closer friendships we have made, the lessons we have learned along the way, the talents we honed on the job, and the wisdom we gleaned as parent or caregiver. Of course, we will also want to keep our loved ones and families, including our church family and the faith it has nurtured down through the years. In other words, as "keepers of meaning" and custodians of the faith, we move to our new home, taking the bones of Joseph with us.

For Further Reading

Barry Baines, *Ethical Wills. Putting Your Values on Paper.* (De Capo Press, 2002.)

William Bridges, *Transitions: Making Sense of Life's Changes,* 2nd edition. (Cambridge, DaCapo Press, 2004.)

Paul C. Clayton, *Called for Life. Finding Meaning in Retirement.* (Herndon Virginia, The Alban Institute, 2008.)

Amy Hanson, *Baby Boomers and Beyond: Tapping the Ministry Talents and Passions of Adults over 50,* 2010. (San Francisco, Jossey-Bass Leadership Network Series, #45, 2010)

David McClelland, *Human Motivation,* (San Francisco, Jossey-Bass Leadership Network Series, #45, 2010.)

John E. Nelson and Richard N. Bolles, *What Color is Your Parachute? For Retirement. Planning a Prosperous, Healthy, and Happy Future.* (Berkeley, the Speed Press, 2010).

Seligman, Martin E. P. *Authentic Happiness. Using New Positive Psychology to Realise Your Potential for Lasting Fulfillment.* (New York, The Free Press, 2002.)

_____, *Flourish. A Visionary Understanding of Happiness and Wellbeing.* (New York, The Free Press, 2011.)

For Viewing

Continue watching and discussing Dewitt Jones, *"For the Love of It."*

Re-Designing Your Life: A Practical Spirituality for the Second Half of Life, Sheila Macdonald Macgregor, Wib Dawson, videographer and editor, 2017.

Questions for Discussion:

Watch Session Five of the videos that have been made to accompany this book and then discuss the following. Note: if you are leading a study group, you may not have time to discuss all the questions. Choose those that you feel will be most helpful to your group.

1. Read Exodus 13. Why do you think Moses carried the bones of Joseph with him when he led the people out of slavery in Egypt? What do we need to carry with us as we move forward into the second half of life?

2. Make a list of those things you want to take with you as you move into your newly renovated house, the things you want

to put in storage for another time, and those things you are ready to discard. What do you notice about the items you have placed in each category?

3. McClelland identifies three major needs that people have: the need for affiliation, the need for power, and the need for achievement. List these needs in your own life. Which would you place first, second, and third in importance for you?

4. Seligman says that there are essentially three approaches to happiness, or three basic ways to be happy: pleasure, engagement, and meaning. Why do we need all three kinds of happiness? Look through various magazines or recall some of the commercials you have seen on television. Which forms of happiness appear most often in the popular media?

Which comes closest to the joy Jesus wants to give us in John 15:11? Why do you think this kind of happiness brings us deep joy, even though we may have suffered tragedy and loss?

5. Amy Hanson recounts an amusing but also powerful story about a very dedicated retired volunteer at her church. What did this man learn from his little granddaughter about the meaning of life? How can the very young teach us important lessons about life and service?

6. What kind of legacy do you want to leave? Consider writing an ethical will to determine your values and whether you are really living them. See Barry Baines's book or visit his website: https://celebrationsoflife.net/ethicalwill-com/.

Chapter 6:
Living in Your New House!

Moving into Your New Home

We are excited because we have just moved into the newly renovated house that is our life. Things seem more satisfying. The pain and sorrow of the Ending we suffered may always be with us, but now it does not colour our whole existence or prevent us from living life to the full. A sense of order replaces the chaos and confusion we experienced in the Neutral Zone. We are ready to make a new Beginning. This does not mean, however, that we will never have to carry out any further renovations. In fact, there is much to be said for doing regular upkeep on the house that is our life.

Repairs and Maintenance

For the first nearly twenty years of our marriage, Richard and I lived in accommodations that we rented, or which were part of my ministry remuneration package. Our first home was a small, furnished, two-room apartment—or "flat," as they call it in Scotland—in a 150-year-old tenement that overlooked a rather grotty canal in an even grottier part of Edinburgh. There was no elevator, just a narrow, crooked staircase with uneven stone steps. Thankfully, we were only on the third floor. The kitchen was just a cupboard in which only one person could work at a time, and there was no real closet space, so Richard had to store his treasured golf clubs beside the toilet. Our only source of heat in the apartment was a tiny heater with a single electric bar. However, we were young and in love, which meant that these things didn't very much matter to us. This was our first home together and it will always have a special place in our hearts. Two more furnished rental homes and three beautiful big church manses later, we finally purchased our own home. By this time, we were of an age when most folks would have had their mortgages paid off. Although we love our home, we quickly discovered that home ownership can have its drawbacks. In the past, when there was a problem with the plumbing or the heating system, we just called the landlord or chairperson of the manse committee and they dealt with it. Now it was up to us to call for professional help—and pay the professional fees!

What we have discovered since we moved into our home nearly fifteen years ago is that it is important to do regular maintenance and repairs. Although I never did the calculations when we started out, I have since learned that the general rule of thumb is that one should anticipate spending roughly three to five percent of the value of your home on repairs and maintenance every year.[163] It sounds like a lot, but the alternative is to let things slide completely and then wind up with an even larger renovations bill.

Just as it is imperative to do regular maintenance work on your house, so also it is important to maintain the home that is your life. In 1 Corinthians 3:16–17, Paul tells us that the body we inhabit is God's

---

163   Romana King, "The ultimate home maintenance guide. A complete schedule of when to do what . . . and how much it costs," *Money Sense*, October 6, 2011.

sacred temple: "Do you not know that you are a temple of God and that the Spirit of God dwells in you? . . . For God's temple is holy, and you are that temple."

Our bodies are sacred. The author of Genesis 1:27 reminds us that we human beings are created in the image and likeness of God. As such, we are called to care for God's image that is our body.

There is a wonderful rabbinic story that illustrates this truth. The famous Rabbi Hillel had just finished a lesson with his students and was making to leave when his pupils asked him where he was going. He replied that he had an important religious duty to perform. He was going off to bathe. One of the pupils ventured to ask for an explanation. "Have you not observed," said he to his disciples, "how the caretakers in the theatres and other public places always wash the statues and keep them clean? If then such care is bestowed on inanimate sculptures, the works of man, it must surely be a holy duty scrupulously to clean the handiwork and masterpiece of God." (Leviticus Rabba 34:3).[164]

Many of us in the second half of life recognise the importance of physical health and commit to a regular exercise program. A large number belong to fitness centres. When I look around my congregation, I am struck by the number of Boomers and older adults who visit the gym two and three times a week or make a point of going for a daily walk to keep in shape.

For example, my friend Liz has always made a point of walking as much as she can. A busy professional woman, Liz works for a major trust company in downtown Toronto. At age sixty, she is tall, slender,

---

164   Address, "Exile and Love," 114.

and beautiful. Her excellent posture and trim figure reflect years of physical activity and good nutrition, giving her an air of self-assurance. She and her seventy-two-year-old husband recently trained for and completed three weeks of hill walking across the north of England and are now heading off on another walking trip through the south of England. Liz radiates good health. Thus no one would guess from her confidence and composure that her number one fear centres on her health. When asked what she would do if she could retire today, she replies without hesitation: "If I were not working right now, I'd really be focussing more on my physical self. [I would be engaging in many] more physical activities. That's what I would be doing right now." Liz recognizes that she has many of the same physical traits and the same body structure as her late mother. Once strong and fit like her daughter, Liz's mother suffered horribly in the final twenty-plus years of her life as her health was greatly diminished by severe osteoporosis.

Like Liz, many of those entering the second half of life are looking at their aging and often ailing parents and gaining a glimpse into what the future may hold for them and, understandably, they are concerned. Rabbi Address states that of the ten major categories in a survey conducted with Jewish baby boomers in the US, the most crucial value that emerged was "health."[165] He adds that maintaining good physical health is entirely in keeping with Jewish teaching. As he notes, good health "allows us to stand in relationship with God" and, as such, is "a powerful tool in our ability to age in a sacred way."[166] When we are sick, or our health is compromised, it can be extremely difficult to focus on matters of the spirit. Quoting the revered mediaeval

---

165   Ibid., 115.

166   Ibid.

Jewish philosopher and physician Rabbi Moses Maimonides, Address observes that maintaining a sound body and vigour has nothing at all to do with today's pursuit of eternal youth, but instead has everything to do with one's ability to serve God. To stay fit, Maimonides recommended "exercise" to "remove the harm caused by most bad habits, which most people have." He also stressed that even "sleep is service to the Almighty."[167]

Closely related to our physical and mental health, of course, is our sexual health. According to a Health Canada survey, "a large majority of people at age sixty-five said that sex was important . . . a majority of those between sixty-five and seventy-four considered themselves sexually active. . . . Sexual activity is a natural and important part of a healthy lifestyle, no matter what your age . . ."[168] Neil Lackey is a registered marriage, family, and sex therapist who practises in Wellesley, Ontario. Our sexuality, he says, is a gift from God, which deserves to be treated with the same care and respect we treat all aspects of our humanity. As we age, we need to have access to safe, trustworthy, and confidential advice on matters related to intimacy and sexuality.

According to Dr. Morris Sherman, chairman of the Canadian Liver Foundation, as more and more boomers re-enter the dating scene after divorce or the death of a spouse, too many are not playing it safe when it comes to sex. Pregnancy—the big fear when practising free love in their youth—is no longer a fear for most of them, and so they erroneously think that they do not need to practise safe sex now. As a consequence, Sherman says that they are seeing more sexually

---

167   Ibid., 116–117.

168   Mila Kadelkova, "Relationships. Understanding the risky sex habits of Canadian baby boomers," *Canadian Living Magazine,* December 3, 2010.

transmitted diseases among boomers than among younger groups.[169] In the church, we think nothing of having discussions on practising safe sex at our youth group meetings or in our young adult ministries. Perhaps it's time we open the discussion up to boomers and older adults and answer their questions with the same respect.

Caring for our physical bodies is how we honour our relationship with God and the image of God within us. The latter, however, represents only one component of good health. Our mental and spiritual health are also vital to establishing a good ecology of health.

Establishing an Ecology of Health

My husband often jokes that he looks forward (many years from now!) to having his obituary printed in our denominational magazine, *The United Church Observer*, which regularly publishes the obituaries of clergy and other church employees and their partners. This is not just because the *Observer* represents religious journalism at its finest; but also because those who wind up in the *Observer's* obits seem to live such long lives.

Dr. Jeff Levin, biomedical scientist, religious scholar, and a pioneer in the field known as the epidemiology of religion, would find nothing surprising in this. While the particular religion does not seem to matter, researchers have found that clergy, and those closely involved in their faith and who attend church regularly, "are forty percent less likely to die of hypertension complicated by heart disease" and, in general, fare much better physically and mentally than those professing no faith.[170] It follows, then, that Richard can expect to enjoy a long life

---

169   Ibid.

170   Jeff Levin, *God, Faith, and Health: Exploring the Spirituality-Healing Connection* (New York: John Wiley & Sons, 2001), 47–56, 60.

simply by virtue of the fact that he accompanies the minister to church every Sunday!

All kidding aside, while affiliation with a religion or membership in a church can never guarantee perfect health or longevity, Levin cites study after study that show that a close connection with religious faith or religious institutions contributes to the maintenance of healthy lifestyles. Not only do many religions encourage healthy behaviour and practices, such as avoidance of smoking, excessive alcohol consumption, and sexual promiscuity, but there are also other religious factors that contribute to sound health. For example, those individuals with strong ties to a faith community reap long-term benefits that extend well beyond spiritual blessings. The positive link between regular attendance at religious services and good health is staggering. Active participation in a community of faith can be a strong support to people undergoing various crises or personal difficulties. As Levin writes, sociological studies affirm that "formal involvement in religious communities reduces the likelihood of experiencing stressors such as chronic and acute illness, marital tension and dissolution, and work-related and legal problems."[171] Faith communities provide people with a good network of friends and thus help to buffer the effects of stress and promote health.[172]

There is also solid evidence to show that participating in worship experiences on a regular basis contributes to feelings of hope, forgiveness, catharsis, and love. My mother was fond of saying that she went to church on Sunday mornings to re-charge her batteries. The worship service gave her a much-needed boost, a sense of comfort, hope, and

---

171　Ibid., 60.
172　Ibid., 61.

joy that carried her through the rest of the week. Little did Mom know then that the positive endorphins she felt after worship, and the boost she got from attending church, have been the subject of numerous well-documented studies.

In addition to more formalized worship experiences, private prayer has also been shown again and again to be a strong determinant of health and well-being. Today, many people talk about "mindfulness," but as Neil Lackey observes, this is just a new way to talk about prayer.[173] It may include liturgical prayer, like confession, petition, and thanksgiving, but goes far beyond the traditional prayers many of us have grown up praying at church.

While not all religious beliefs are created equal and bad religion, too, often leads to feelings of guilt, anger, diminished self-esteem, and depression, healthy religious beliefs can and frequently do contribute to good mental health. This was the finding of Duke University psychiatrist Dr. Harold G. Koenig in his book *Aging and God*. Especially as we age, our faith may help us to cope better with existing illness and provide some relief from mental health challenges like depression, anxiety, and thoughts of suicide.[174] Indeed, as Levin notes, "a study of eighty-five older Canadians found that high scores on a Christian "orthodoxy scale" were associated with greater happiness and life satisfaction."[175] Religious beliefs, it would seem, enhance our sense of self-esteem and contribute to positive feelings of self-worth.

---

173   Interview with Neil Lackey, Wellesley, ON, September 16, 2016.

174   William M. Clements and Harold G. Koenig, *Aging and God: Spiritual Pathways to Mental Health in Midlife and Later Years* (London: Routledge, 1994); Levin, *God, Faith, and Health*, 93.

175   Levin, *God, Faith, and Health*, 100.

Faith is not a magic bullet when it comes to maintaining good physical and mental health, but there is ample evidence to suggest that it can be a powerful tool in preventing or lessening the negative effects of illness.[176] Simply put, this is because faith leads "to thoughts of hope, optimism, and positive expectation."[177] Employing Paul's language in *Ephesians 6:11,* Levin says that faith and hope are "an integral part of the 'whole armour of God'" and, as such, they can help to "shield someone, at least in part, from the harmful effects of stressful circumstances."[178] Indeed, the healing balm provided by feelings of hopefulness is by far the most important way that religious faith impacts health. Quoting Koenig's foundational research with older adults, Levin writes:

> [Religious faith] provides a mechanism by which attitudes can be changed and life circumstances reframed. . . . The degree of hope and emotional strength afforded by religion to some older adults may far exceed that obtainable from other sources.[179]

It is perhaps no accident therefore that the longevity revolution parallels the spirituality wave. Boomers, for whom health is the number-one concern, are discovering that the faith many of them abandoned back in the sixties and seventies may well provide the key to better physical and mental health, and that a vibrant spirituality, nurtured

---

176   Levin is also careful to point out that "the illness, suffering, or death of a particular person in no way should be—or can be—attributed to a lack of faith or not enough spirituality." "Epidemiology is incapable of addressing such issues. What it can tell us—and does very clearly—is that religious involvement deserves to be recognized as one of the significant factors that promotes health and well-being among groups of people." Ibid., 8.

177   Ibid., 144.

178   Ibid., 150.

179   Ibid., 137.

by a caring community, is central to a healthy ecology of body, mind, and spirit. Levin identifies this as the "theosomatic medical model."[180] However we choose to name this, it is clear that there is more involved in achieving well-being than just good genes, luck, or even exercise and sound nutrition, however important the latter may be. A deepening relationship to God, our higher self, and our fellow travellers on the spiritual journey contribute immeasurably to our overall health because together they bring us hope.

Friendship and Hope

As we have seen, hope is central to health and well-being. It allows people to reframe an illness or a difficult or demoralizing situation and to look at things in a more positive light. University of Aberdeen professor of theology John Swinton argues that "a key to such reframing of illness experience and the instillation of hope lies in friendship."[181] He asserts, moreover, that Jesus and the model of friendship he espoused can help to bring healing to people facing sickness and depression. His findings are supported by David Bieble and Harold Koenig, who write that "healing . . . can only occur within the context of supportive relationships."[182]

To this day, one of my favourite hymns is "What A Friend We Have in Jesus." Years later, I learned that this was actually my Grandmother Crombie's favourite hymn. I wonder if she sang it to herself when she

---

180   Ibid., 207-222, 251.

181   John Swinton, *Resurrecting the Person: Friendship and the Care of People with Mental Health Problems* (Nashville: Abingdon Press, 2000), 138.

182   David E. Bieble and Harold C. Koenig, *New Light on Depression: Help, Hope and Answers for the Depressed and Those Who Love Them* (Grand Rapids: Zondervan, 2004), Location 3938.

was feeling so homesick for her family back in beautiful Ireland that first winter in the French River. It was a hymn we sang every week at CGIT (Canadian Girls in Training—Explorers) and Pioneer Girls. Overweight and afflicted by a particularly virulent case of acne, I suffered very low self-esteem during my pre-pubescent and adolescent years. I realise now that I was probably not alone and that many young people find this a challenging period. However, for me, knowing that I had a friend in Jesus, one who loved me "spots and all," was a great comfort. Jesus's words in John 15:15, which we were encouraged to memorize, continue to be for me some of the most beautiful words I have ever heard and I cherish them: "No longer do I call you servants, for the servant does not know what his master is doing; but I have called you friends, for all that I have heard from my Father I have made known to you." (ESV)

When we observe the friendships of Jesus, the first thing that strikes us is his ability to be able to see the whole person, the person behind the sin, the sickness, or the spots. By sharing friendship with the broken, the lonely or isolated, the marginalized or shunned, Jesus was able to restore them to "wholeness," to reinstate them to their rightful place in God's community and give them hope. In Luke 19:1–10, Jesus spies the hated tax collector Zacchaeus hiding in the branches of a sycamore tree and, instead of shunning him, which was the expected treatment for those who collected taxes for the reviled Roman government, Jesus told Zacchaeus to come down so that Jesus could visit with him at his home that very day. The crowd was shocked that Jesus, a Jew, would sully himself by being a guest of a tax collector. Likewise, Jesus's disciples were shocked when they discovered him visiting with a Samaritan woman in John 4. But Jesus was able to see beyond all those things that stigmatized her and kept her an outcast. Her gender, race, and questionable personal morality were not barriers for Jesus. He was able to see her for who she was and listen to her story, just as he had listened to Zacchaeus and many others. By drinking from the cup she offered him, Jesus not only takes on her limitations and sinfulness, but he also makes it possible for her to be restored to full standing in the family of God. As Swinton writes, "in doing this, he takes her into the community of God, resurrects her personhood, and heals her brokenness."[183] Even with the Garasene man (Luke 8), ostracized from the community because he was purported to have been possessed by demons, Jesus shows incredible compassion and respect. It is significant that in healing him and, later, the ten lepers, in Luke 17, the first thing Jesus does is to send them back to their community—to restore them to their family and friends. Jesus knew that wholeness and healing depend to a large degree on being in relationship with others.[184]

Again, it's important to note the nature of Jesus's friendships. Swinton writes:

> Jesus's friendships were always personal, as opposed to instrumental, primarily aimed at regaining the dignity and personhood of those whom society had rejected and depersonalized. Jesus's friendships reached beyond the socially constructed identity of individuals and, in entering into deep and personal relationships of friend- ship with them, he was able to reveal something of the

---

183   Swinton, *Resurrecting the Person*, 142.

184   As we have already seen, this was one of the major findings from Vaillant's research with the men of the Harvard Grant Study. Relationships are central to health and happiness, especially in old age.

> nature of God and enable the development of a posi-
> tive sense of personhood based on intrinsic value rather
> than on personal achievement or outward behaviour. .
> . . the friendships of Jesus reached beyond social expec-
> tations to reclaim the personhood of the other. This
> type of friendship is catalytic.[185]

While committed friendship is not a substitute for prescribed medication and psychotherapy treatments, it can greatly aid in the recovery
process. This is because one of the primary ways people find hope is
through caring, supportive interpersonal relationships. Medication
and therapy may be necessary, but understanding brings another powerful dimension to the healing process that should not be discounted
and which is probably the best gift that brothers and sisters in the
faith community can bring to one who is suffering. What this means
is taking the time to really listen to the person who is hurting, to value
that individual as a whole person and not simply as someone who
suffers from a physical or mental illness. It means not only accept-
ing the individual's perspective on his or her own suffering, but, more
importantly, being willing also to accept that person for who he or she
is.[186] Again, I can't emphasize enough the importance of really listening
to the one who suffers.

A light-hearted story illustrates what I mean. In their book *Stories of
the Spirit*, Jack Kornfield and Christina Feldman share this story:

> A family went out to a restaurant for dinner. When
> the waitress arrived, the parent gave their orders.

---

185   Swinton, *Resurrecting the Person*, 142-143.
186   Ibid., 141.

Immediately, the five-year-old daughter piped up with her own: "I'll have a hot dog, French fries, and a Coke." "Oh, no, you won't," interjected the dad and, turning to the waitress, he said, "She'll have meatloaf, mashed potatoes, and milk." Looking at the child with a smile, the waitress said, "So, hon, what do want on that hot dog?" When she left, the family sat stunned and silent. A few moments later the little girl, eyes shining, said, "She thinks I'm real."[187]

In my own life, I know that when I have been feeling down or discouraged, it is to my friends that I often turn for care and support. I know I can count on them to listen to my thoughts. Enjoying a cup of tea or coffee with a close friend can help me to put my situation into perspective. I have found, too, that regular heartfelt sharing and a few laughs over lunch with my long-time friend Deb, or a phone conversation with my cousin Patti in Edmonton, are the finest forms of preventive medicine I know. I often tell our pastoral visitors at Siloam that the best thing they can do for the shut-ins they visit is to be a friend: to really listen to the person and affirm his or her story. As Swinton notes, Christ-like friendship is catalytic in nature. Unlike the more instrumental relationships, which doctors and therapists provide, it does not aim to do anything: "It is a form of relationship that acts as a catalyst that enables health and re-humanization simply by being there."[188] People who are lonely or suffering from ill health, especially poor mental health, don't need yet another person to do anything for

---

187 Quoted in Tara Brack, *Growing Up Unworthy*, April 19, 2012; Jack Kornfield and Christina Feldman, *Stories of the Spirit* (San Francisco: Harper, 1991).

188 Swinton, *Resurrecting the Person*, 43.

them. What they need is someone to be their friend, to be there for them when they need a listening ear or a shoulder to cry on, someone who accompanies them on their journey.

Neil Lackey tells of two ministries that his former congregation, St. Paul's United in Milverton, Ontario, implemented years ago that have been very successful. The first was called simply "Friends." People in the congregation volunteered to visit the housebound in the community, just to offer a friendly visit. Often the health unit would call and ask if a visit could be made to one of their clients. No clergy were involved, except in a supportive role to the visitors. The UCW ladies at my former congregation in Thorndale, Ontario, continue to provide this ministry, as do many UCW groups throughout Canada.

The second ministry that Neil's congregation engaged in evolved out of the Friends program. This was a kind of help line—at first primarily for seniors, but which later came to include all people. The purpose was to provide basic support and helpful contact information and resources that people could access through one centralized phone number. Again, this ministry enabled people to share Christ's friendship with those in the wider community and accompany people on their journey.

The gift of accompaniment is one that many in the second half of life are able to offer. With years of lived experience behind us, the time afforded by retirement, and mostly good health, we have an opportunity to accompany those who often live with stigmatization due to mental illness or who wrestle with loneliness and disabilities.

The Gift of Accompaniment

In her very helpful book, *Jewish Vision for Aging*, Rabbi Dayle Friedman cites an interesting conversation she had with her colleague in ministry, Rabbi Margaret Holub. Holub has served as a rabbi with homeless people, both within her congregation and on the streets. The job of the rabbi, she believes, is one of *livui ruchani*, spiritual accompaniment. Again, more than actually doing anything, and "more than fixing or changing people, our job, she says, is to walk along with people through the sorrows, joys, and everyday moments of their lives."[189] This ministry of presence or accompaniment is also the vocation of all who seek to offer friendship in the name of that other great rabbi, Jesus.

Without knowing it, perhaps, many mature adults engage in the ministry of accompaniment, using these extra years that have been given them to visit nursing homes, retirement centres, hospices, prisons, homeless shelters, as well as people who live alone in their own homes. Along with the gifts of friendship and presence, Friedman identifies two qualities that can help people in their ministry of accompaniment: humility and respect.[190] Whether we are visiting the very elderly, the sick, or the homeless, it is important we treat people with dignity, and not like helpless infants. (Even the use of such terms as "the elderly," "the sick," and "the homeless" can be very demeaning!) This is a special challenge in caring for frail, older adults, particularly our parents. Friedman reminds us that the bible admonishes us to respect our

---

189   Rabbi Dayle Friedman, *Jewish Visions for Aging: A Professional Guide for Fostering Wholeness. Text and Tradition. Aging and Meaning. Family Caregiving. Livui Ruchani: Spiritual Accompaniment in Aging. Aging and Community.* (Woodstock, VT: Jewish Lights Publishing), 121.

190   Ibid., 120.

elders: "Rise before the gray-haired, and grant glory to the face of the elder" (Leviticus 19:32).

Caregiving: Honouring Our Fathers and Mothers

When I was in seminary at Princeton back in the early eighties, one of my student internships was at the local nursing home. There, I met people who could remember starring in local amateur theatrical productions with the likes of Hollywood superstar Jimmy Stewart, who once studied engineering at Princeton. Many of these people were very witty and sharp and had wonderful stories to tell. Their limitations were more physical in nature. A remark made to me in passing one day by an elderly African American woman who was wheelchair bound was very telling and has always stayed with me. That afternoon was movie day and, for the umpteenth time, the well-meaning activities director had brought in another travelogue. The woman turned to me and said, "I don't mind watching travel shows, but I wish they would show other films, too. It's as if they are afraid to show us any of the newer releases for fear that we won't be able to handle it, that it will be too shocking for us." In trying to protect her residents, the activities director forgot that these older people were once young themselves, that they had seen a lot of life, and should have been allowed to engage as fully in life as they were able, including being able to make their own decisions about what they watched during movie time.

This tendency to want to protect the most senior members of our community presents itself in other areas, particularly around personal safety issues. It is perhaps natural for adult children to want to protect their elderly parents and avoid all situations that involve risk in order to keep them safe, but being able to make choices and take risks are part of what it means to be human. Unless there is clear evidence to indicate that the person is not capable of making decisions, he or she should be allowed to decide what level of risk is comfortable. This is what the "differently abled" advocates refer to as the "dignity of risk." In addition to allowing our parents the freedom to take risks and even to fail, it is important that we do not rob them of opportunities to serve or make a contribution, for it is through serving that people experience meaning and joy.

I always remember staying with the ninety-nine-year-old mother-in-law of one of my seminary professors while he and his wife went away for a weekend. Mrs. Pentecost was frail and nearly blind, but as much as possible, she maintained her independence in the attic apartment where she lived in her daughter's home. I was in the home just to make sure that she got regular meals, but she was able to dress herself, manage the bathroom and even the stairs that led down to the kitchen. Her daughter raised canaries, and I recall that their care was far more intricate than looking after Mrs. Pentecost! However, I wasn't alone in caring for the birds. Mrs. Pentecost would spend hours each day shredding bits of fabric, remnants from her daughter's sewing basket, and the shredded fabric was placed in the birdcages so that the birds could build their nests. It was a small and rather tedious task, but it gave the elderly Mrs. Pentecost a purpose and made her feel like she was contributing to the household—which, of course, she was. It also allowed her to maintain her dignity.

Questions about how to care with dignity for elderly parents, and sometimes partners have become a major theme of those entering the second half of life. There is no question that the "age wave" has created a parallel "caregiving wave." According to Canadian retirement coach Janet Christensen, "statistically in North America, seventy-five percent of the population at some point in their life will have elder-care issues and responsibilities. . . . Right now at any given time, twenty-five percent of the population is currently engaged in elder care."[191] Christensen notes that this has serious financial implications, particularly for women because women are more likely to leave their jobs in order to care for an elderly parent or relative. Keeping in mind that many of these same women left the workforce for maternity leaves or to spend time raising their children, this means that not only their career and potential earnings have been adversely affected, but so also have their pensions. Even with the adjustment that CPP makes for women who took time out to have children, women still take more of a financial hit for time missed caring for family and this affects their ability to have a decent retirement. On a personal note, a friend of mine found that she had to take a major cut in her pension when she retired just two years early from her teaching career to care for her ailing mother.

Many people in my congregation find themselves running back and forth to doctors' appointments with their loved ones. Some of these people need to work full-time, and others still have teenage children to provide for, at least financially. In some cases, adult children have moved back home, sometimes bringing with them grandchildren who need even more attention. One couple in my congregation has had to wrestle with one partner's health concerns while making daily trips to another city to tend to an aged parent struggling with the recent death of a spouse and her own ill health. At one point, the wife was running between hospitals in two different cities to visit her husband

---

191   Janet Christensen interview.

and mother. Many suffer from economic, emotional, professional, and physical exhaustion, combined with feelings of guilt. Just when they most need to be able to nurture their own physical, emotional, and spiritual well-being, they find they have no time for themselves. In addition, differences of opinion among siblings as to how best to care for Dad or Mom, sometimes from well-meaning relatives who live far away from the one who is providing the primary care, may awaken family conflicts that have lain dormant for years.[192]

It can be especially hard if the one you are caring for is your partner, particularly if there seems to be little possibility of improved health for this person you have promised to love and cherish all your life. Susan is a fifty-six-year-old registered nurse from the small rural community of Tara, near Owen Sound, Ontario. She and her husband Larry have been married thirty-eight years and have two adult sons and two adult daughters, all of whom are married with young children of their own. Nine years ago, things looked promising for a happy retirement. With the kids grown and on their own, Susan and Larry were looking forward to the day when they could step back from their respective careers in nursing and farming and spend more time in their golden years travelling, enjoying the grandchildren, and doing some of the things they had always dreamed of doing together. Then, at the age of fifty, Larry had a serious farm accident, which left him a quadriplegic. Their dreams were shattered. There would be no winter holidays in Florida, nor even long walks along the beaches of nearby Lake Huron.

To this day, Larry remains on a ventilator, a prisoner of his wheelchair. Susan works long hours at the South Bruce Grey Health Centre in

---

192   Friedman, *Jewish Visions for Aging*, 71-74.

Chesley. She expects that she will need to keep working full-time until she is at least sixty-eight because she desperately needs the benefits her job provides to care for Larry. Nearly all her pay goes to providing full-time care for Larry when she is working, as the government provides her with only a very limited number of homecare hours so that she can get her groceries and tend to household chores and other necessary business. Since the farm insurance did not provide them with much, they were left with very little money to purchase the high-powered $21,000 wheelchair that Larry requires or to carry out the extensive renovations they had to make to their farmhouse to accommodate his needs. None of the major hospitals or health centres will provide them with even respite care because they feel that Larry's needs are too extensive. Moreover, because a certain level of training is required to attend to his needs, it is not possible for even a neighbour to slip over for a while and give Susan a break. Indeed, many of their friends have stopped visiting because they don't know what to say anymore.

For Susan, the nights are long and she seldom gets the rest she needs. While she once enjoyed her job, now it has become more of a means to an end, as she focuses on her primary goal of providing care to Larry. She doesn't complain because she knows that things are far worse for him and that he frequently suffers from depression. Since life was too busy before Larry's accident, there did not seem to be enough time to participate in a local congregation of faith to nurture their spirit or build the important relationships that a faith community can often provide. The Mennonites were good to them in the beginning, but now they have no spiritual support to carry them. The golden years have turned out to be nothing but a cruel joke. This is not how they had hoped to spend the second half of life. Susan's advice to others is to "prepare for the very worst!" As she says, if they had had more savings, life today would be a bit more comfortable for Larry and certainly much easier for her.[193] For now, she does everything she can to help him maintain his personal dignity and keep him in the family home, even though it comes at a huge cost to her own well-being. This is a true living out of the wedding vows "for better, for worse; for richer, for poorer; in sickness and in health."

Susan and Larry's story speaks to the complexity, loneliness, and intensity of suffering often inherent in caregiving relationships. But clearly, their story is not uncommon. Wendy Haaf writes that "according to the Statistics Canada report "Family Caregivers: What Consequences?" in 2012, eight million of us were providing unpaid care for a friend or family member—that's nearly one in three."[194] As she adds, "of those informal caregivers, twenty percent were aged fifty-five to sixty-four and twelve percent were sixty-five or older."[195] How do we provide compassion and support for the caregiver, while at the same time ministering to the needs of the one requiring our love and care? Friedman writes that our loved ones must be respected and valued. Yet, as she points out, there is nothing in the biblical tradition that insists "that we must be consumed by caregiving, wrung dry, and left with nothing for ourselves and our own families."[196] There are no easy answers to these situations. One thing, however, is sure. Caregivers must look after themselves if they are to be helpful to those for whom they are caring. I often liken this to the instructions one is given regarding the use of

---

193　Conversation with Susan Galbraith, September 4, 2016.

194　Wendy Haaf, "A User's Guide for Caregivers," *Good Times. Canada's Magazine for Successful Retirement.* December 2016, 19–23.

195　Ibid.

196　Friedman, *Jewish Visions for Aging*, 104.

oxygen masks on an aircraft. Just as one needs to adjust one's own mask before attempting to help someone else, so, also, do caregivers need to care for themselves before trying to help others. Indeed, caregivers will need to draw upon all their resources, including spiritual resources, in order to meet these still relatively new twenty-first-century challenges.

Sharing the Ministry of Friendship and Accompaniment

Perhaps the best way we can be supportive of both sufferer and care-giver is to share in the ministry of friendship and accompaniment. As Haaf and others point out, maintaining good social connections is paramount for both caregiver and the one being cared for. Even as Jesus prepared for death on the cross, he found time to be with, to listen to, and to commune with his friends (Matthew 26:26). By affirming the stories of sufferer and caregiver, we model the friendship of Jesus and help to restore them to full community in the family of God. By sharing Jesus's stories, we bring hope to the broken in spirit and good news to the afflicted. At Siloam, we share this commission every Sunday at the close of worship: "Let us go out to fulfill our high calling as servants and friends of Jesus Christ that we may be Christ to each other and God's world." To be sure, we do not carry out this mission alone, but rather as members of the community of faith. As Friedman writes, "it takes a village to raise a child; so, too, may we come to realise that it takes an entire community to care for frail elders [and partners] and their caregivers."[197]

A beautiful story recounted by Father William Bausch speaks to our need for community, especially when we are hurting. Bausch writes:

---

197   Ibid., 81.

A woman's happiness was shattered by the loss of her brother, a good man, dearly loved. Torn by anguish, she kept asking God, "Why?" But hearing only silence, she set out in search of an answer. She had not gone far when she came upon an old man sitting on a bench. He was weeping. He said, "I have suffered a great loss. I am a painter, and I have lost my eyesight." He, too, was seeking an answer to the question, "Why?" The woman invited him to join her and, taking him by the arm, they trudged down the road.

Soon, they overtook a young man walking aimlessly. He had lost his wife, the source of his joy, to another man. He joined in the search of an answer to the "why" question. Shortly, they came upon a young woman weeping on her front doorstep. She had lost her child. She, too, joined them. Nowhere could they find an answer.

Suddenly, they came upon Jesus Christ. Each confronted him with their questions, but Jesus gave no answer. Instead, he began to cry and said, "I am bearing the burden of a woman who has lost her brother, a young mother whose child has died, a painter who has lost his eyesight, and a young man who has lost a love in which he delighted." As he spoke, the four moved closer, and they embraced each other. And they grasped Jesus's hands.

Jesus spoke again, saying, "My dominion is the dominion of the heart. I cannot prevent pain. I can only heal it." "How?" asked the woman. "By sharing it," he said. And then he was gone. And the four? They were left standing, holding each other.[198]

Telling Your Story: Writing Your Autobiography

An important part of the ministry of accompaniment is the ability not only to be able to hold each other close, but also to hold one another's stories. Listening, as we have seen, is how we affirm others and share friendship.

Years ago, when I was in parish ministry in Edinburgh, Scotland, I had a lovely visit with an older member of my congregation. Her name was Jennie Somerville, and she was the younger sister of the famous Christian missionary and runner, Eric Liddell. You may remember seeing his story, which was portrayed in the wonderful movie, *Chariots of Fire.*

Known as "the flying Scotsman," Eric was born in China, the son of Scottish missionaries. He returned to Edinburgh to study for the ministry. While he was at New College Divinity School, he had an opportunity to enter the 1924 Olympics, which were being hosted by the City of Paris. Eric was a committed Christian and refused to race on a Sunday, with the consequence that he was forced to withdraw from the 100-metre race, his best event. Up until then, he was the darling of Scotland. After he refused to run on a Sunday, he was greatly ridiculed

---

198   William J. Bausch, *A World of Stories for Preachers and Teachers* (Mystic, CT: Twenty-Third Publications, 1998), 274.

and condemned by the British press. In the end, Eric competed in the 400-metre race, which was not scheduled for a Sunday. Just as he was about to start the race, someone came up to him and slipped a piece of paper into his hand with a quotation from 1 Samuel 2:30, *"Those who honour me I will honour."* Liddell ran with that piece of paper in his hand. He not only won the race but broke the existing world record with a time of 47.6 seconds.

That part of the story is true. What is not true is the way that Eric's sister Jennie was portrayed in that film. If you recall the movie, you will know that Jennie was portrayed as a prim, down-in-the-mouth killjoy, who was very critical of Eric and his athletic aspirations. She was constantly nagging her brother, telling him that he needed to focus more on his theological studies and less on his running. According to the film, she didn't want Eric to run in the Olympics. In point of fact, nothing could have been further from the truth. Jennie was just a little girl living in China with her parents at the time Eric ran in the Paris Olympics. Not only would she not have opposed his race, the fact is that she didn't even know about it until long after it was over. Indeed, she and her parents did not learn that Eric had even entered the Olympics until months after he had won the gold medal! Moreover, she was always very proud of her older brother. But the director of the film told Jennie that he needed a point of tension in the film, and since he couldn't pin any sexual scandal on Eric, he chose to have his character interact with a very negative and fictitious older sister. Thus, Jennie Somerville's character was horribly maligned. And yet she was such a lovely, happy, gracious, and kind lady! I promised her that wherever I went—and whenever I had the opportunity—I would tell her story as it should have been told.

Writing your life story enables you to tell your story as it should be told, from the perspective of the one who—apart from God—knows you best. By revisiting your personal story, you also have an opportunity to re-examine emotional baggage that you may have been carrying around for years. Once you have a chance to put things in perspective, you may find it less significant than you previously imagined. A real bonus is that you may also develop closer friendships with siblings and other family members as you share stories from your childhood. Capturing a personal or family history can even help resolve old family conflicts and enable family members to understand each other better. Grandparents who want to leave their grandchildren a powerful legacy will be interested to learn that studies carried out at Emory University reveal that families who share their family history have kids who have greater self-esteem and do better academically.

For those who are engaged in caring for an elderly relative, life review can be a powerful tool in assisting the one who needs care. This is what Friedman calls "sacred listening."[199] By listening to another's story, you honour that individual. Such listening also goes a long way toward creating a safe space for both the caregiver and the one receiving the care to express emotions without feeling that they are being judged. It is natural to experience some distress when we watch the decline of those we have loved and looked up to all our lives. Inviting them to share their story with us can provide an antidote to the sorrow we may feel by allowing us to consider what in this person's story we can hold on to and focus on the blessing their life has been. What is their legacy to us?

---

199   Friedman, *Jewish Visions for Aging*, 120–123, 135.

These are not the only benefits to reviewing your life story. Several recent scientific studies have shown that talking about your life experiences lowers blood pressure and strengthens the immune system. Plus, there is a wealth of anecdotal evidence in the published scientific literature that affirms that "life review" is of tremendous help to people experiencing grief. Not only does it lower levels of depression, but it is also found to increase problem-solving skills and self-esteem while assisting in the grief process.[200]

Another helpful exercise, as we saw in our last chapter, is based on an ancient spiritual tradition that is also found in the Hebrew and Christian scriptures. This is the creation of an ethical will or what is sometimes called a legacy letter. Writing an ethical will or legacy letter is also good practice for writing your life story or memoirs. Many people find it easier to start with an ethical will before tackling the more daunting task of writing a full-scale autobiography. You may find that it is one of the most cherished and meaningful gifts you can give to your loved ones, too!

Gratitude: Rounding Out the Ecology of Health

Writing an ethical will or personal memoir is also one of the best gifts you can give yourself, especially in this time of transition. By engaging in life review, either by writing an ethical will or autobiography, you have an opportunity to reflect on where you have been, what has been life-giving for you, what you need to discard to move forward, and what you now need to keep in order to create a life of meaning.

allows you to celebrate your life and give thanks to God for

ennebaker, *Opening Up: The Healing Power of Expressing Emotions*
· The Guilford Press, 1997.)

the blessings you have known and the opportunities that lie ahead. Gratitude rounds out the ecology of health we seek to create. According to psychology professor Robert Emmons, when you practise gratitude on a daily basis, you are healthier physically, mentally, and spiritually.[201] It not only reduces stress and helps to create a better and stronger immune system, but also helps you to look at life from a more positive perspective. You begin to see the world from the vantage point of "the glass half full," rather than "half empty." As we build the house that we want to inhabit in the second half of life, we can do no better therefore than to start with the foundation of thanksgiving.[202] As Izaak Walton once said: "God has two dwellings—one in heaven, and the other in a meek and thankful heart."[203]

Ritual as an Orientating Anchor

It is not uncommon for people to have housewarming parties when they move into a new home. Sometimes, we will have an open house to celebrate the completion of an addition or recently renovated room. Although the job of maintenance and repair is always ongoing, there are nevertheless times when it is appropriate to celebrate the changes we have made to our living space. The same is true of the home we call our life.

A ritual that had great meaning for some of the members in my home congregation centred around identifying what we need to let go of as we transition into the second half of life and what we need to keep.

---

201   Trisha Elliott, The Gratitude Effect, *The United Church Observer*, October 2016, pp. 24-27.

202   Friedman, *Jewish Visions for Aging*, 172-173.

203   Mark Link SJ, *100 Stories for Special Occasion Homilies*, (Allen, Texas, Tabor Publishing, 1992), p. 60.

Each member brought two small objects, one that symbolized "letting go" and another that symbolized "holding close."[204] After speaking about the significance of each item, members placed them on the communion table around which we afterwards celebrated the Lord's Supper together. It was a very meaningful act and one that had emotional resonance for those involved.

It reminded me of an experience I had had years earlier, on my tenth birthday. My paternal grandmother, then aged eighty-six, invited me to her place for lunch. She knew that my friends and I loved to have tea parties, and so she set her dining room table with her best linens, china, and silverware, adorned it with a crystal and silver vase in which she placed a single rose, and asked me to sit with her and offer grace. We enjoyed tea and scones with jam and had a lovely afternoon together. Grannie shared stories about growing up on the farm in Craigleith, near Collingwood, Ontario, and how she used to have to snowshoe to school in the winter. She talked about studying music in Edinburgh when she was in her twenties, about her studies in home economics in the 1890s at what is now the University of Guelph, how she met and married my grandfather, and how she took my four-year-old father on a trip to meet his father in France, where his father had served as a medical doctor in World War I. Apparently, they hit an iceberg off the coast of Newfoundland just a couple of hours into their voyage. As this was only a few years after the sinking of the Titanic, everyone was terrified. But they managed to make it back safely to shore and, eventually, to set sail again for Europe, this time successfully. It was a beautiful journey down memory lane. When our visit ended, my grandmother told me that everything on the table was now mine. It was her birthday

---

204   Thanks to group member Richard Graham for this suggestion.

present to me. Looking back on that afternoon, I realise that what we shared in was a sacred moment, a true sacrament of love and grace. There was the chalice (teapot), the breaking of bread (the scones and jam), there was scripture (the memories that were shared), and there was prayer. Not too long after this, my grandmother gave up her home and moved into a seniors' residence. This ritual marked her leaving the home where she had lived following the untimely death of her husband some thirty years earlier.

In her book, Friedman recounts a somewhat similar tale about "leaving home," or transitioning into a new phase of life. She talks about Carol and Bob, who had decided to "downsize" from the large family home where they had raised their children and lived for forty-three years. Because they had shared so many memories with family and friends in this home, they decided to mark the transition to a smaller home with a special celebration. So they gathered their children and grand-children around the dining room table for a special dinner. Everyone shared memories of the times they had spent in that house. There were happy memories, and there were sad ones. All of them were included. Later, Bob and Carol and one of their adult children went through the entire house, sharing memories specific to each room. They finished by sharing a prayer of gratitude for all the good things they had experienced in the house and for those good things that were still to come. Once they made the move, they held another party with close friends to celebrate their transition into the new home. Carol said afterward that this ritual helped to ease the pain of leaving a home that had filled their lives with memory, so much so that she found she was able to move forward contentedly and begin to create new memories.[205]

---

205   Ibid.

One of the sad things about moving into the second half of life is that there is such a dearth of ritual to mark our experiences. One of the joys of moving into the second half of life is that we now can create new rituals to frame our experiences, just as Carol and Bob did; just as my grandmother did with me years ago.

As Friedman and many others have noted, "ritual can serve as an orienting anchor" when we are faced with change or loss.[206] It can give us a sense of stability and continuity when our lives are in flux or when we are confused about the direction we should now follow. At the funeral or memorial service, it can affirm meaning in the face of death by giving the grieving widow or widower an opportunity to celebrate the life of a beloved partner, while at the same time affirming that those who mourn are held within the love of God and the care of the surrounding community. Ritual can connect us to past events in our lives, while helping us to appreciate the present and look forward to the future. Now that we are living much longer than previous generations, there needs to be more than just the traditional retirement lunch and funeral service to mark our years. There needs to be rites of passage to celebrate the birth of grandchildren, the assumption of a new volunteer role, the undertaking of a new religious study or practice, the onset of menopause, the entering of a new community, or the beginning of a new romantic relationship. For example, those who experience the death of a spouse or the end of a marriage through divorce do not always want to enter another marriage. Yet, they may have found a new love that brings their lives meaning and joy in the second half. What are the ethical and religious implications of such a relationship, which is now more common than ever? Should we be

---

206   Ibid.

creating rituals to honour these new relationships? And, if so, how do we do this in a way that continues to uphold the sanctity of marriage and yet recognizes the new relationship?

How do we mark more negative experiences in our lives? It is hard to live with a disability, to lose a friend, or become the caregiver to an incapacitated parent or partner. It is difficult to be given bad news about your health, or to be told that you or your loved one now requires full-time nursing home care. When my brother William and I buried our widowed father, he turned to me and said: "Well, Sheila, we are now orphans," even though we were well into the second half of life. It was a strange feeling. We were now our own front line. Apart from the service to celebrate my father's life, there was nothing to mark this new phase into which William and I had entered.

Separation and divorce can be particularly hard as we enter the second half of life, but they are becoming a common feature of this period. Among all the generations, in fact, boomers now have the highest rate of divorce. We even have a name for this phenomenon. It's called *grey divorce,* and it is on the rise even in Canada. In June of 2016, *Zoomer Magazine* reported that, in Canada, divorce is sparking among the fifty-pluses and becoming an increasingly common event for couples aged sixty-five and older.[207] As a result, loneliness among boomers is also on the rise.

How do we acknowledge the pain that is always involved in such decisions, regardless of whether it is a break-up that has been agreed upon by both parties? One couple chose to engage in a ritual in which they

---

207   Wendy Dennis, "How Grey Divorce Became the New Normal," *Zoomer Magazine,* June 3, 2016.

buried the wedding veil in the ground. However, if one partner did not want the divorce—or if that person left the marriage for someone else—there is the danger that more than the veil might wind up buried in the earth, possibly strangled by and shrouded in the very veil that had once been part of a ceremony of love and celebration! This, of course, simply highlights the need for our rituals to be sensitive to the feelings of those involved, to have credibility, and to be grounded in community.

Rabbi Richard Address, founder and director of Jewish Sacred Aging, believes strongly in the importance of ritual for the second half of life.[208] Drawing on the wisdom of his Jewish colleagues, Address has created a website that provides a large selection of rituals and prayers for some of the new life situations facing those in the second half of life. Not only are there rituals for retirement and milestone birthdays and anniversaries, but there are also resources that he and others have created to mark such sacred moments as leaving one's family home, removing one's wedding ring on the first anniversary of a spouse's death, receiving a diagnosis of Alzheimer's disease, entering a hospice, removing a loved one from life support, or coming out later in life to one's family or community as gay, lesbian, or transgendered.[209] There are even rituals to bless the union of couples where one or both partners has a spouse who is suffering from dementia and no longer knows them. These individuals do not wish to divorce their marriage partners, whom they promised to love in sickness and in health; but at the same

---

208   Rabbi Richard Address, Theme Speaker at the 7th International Conference on Ageing and Spirituality at Concordia University (Chicago), June 4 to 7, 2017.

209   Sheila Macgregor, "Marking the Meaning in Grieving, Coming Out, Diagnosis, Birthdays, Co-habitating. Why this stage of life needs its own rituals in *Zoomer Magazine*, everythingzoomer.com, October 2017.

time they are struggling to find a way to honour a new relationship that has brought their life joy and meaning.

Again, we come back to the centrality of community. Rituals are valuable because they remind us of our connectedness to God and to others—those who have gone before us, those who share our lives now, and those yet unborn. They remind us that we are never alone and that our existence and life have meaning. Craig Miller, who has studied boomers for over two decades and written extensively on boomer spirituality, says that loneliness is one of the most pervasive features of boomer life stories and one to which the church needs to pay serious attention.[210] Rituals that celebrate our common journey and link us more closely with the faith community can bring deep personal enrichment and point the way to the mystery that is God.

For Further Reading

Anne Beattie-Stokes, *A Heart of Wisdom. Inspiration and Instruction for Conscious Elderhood.* (North Charleston, SC, Booksurge Publishing, 2009.)

Richard Address, *Seekers of Meaning. Baby Boomers, Judaism, and the Pursuit of Healthy Aging.* (New York, URJ Press, 2012.)

Joan Chittister, *The Gift of Years. Growing Older Gracefully.* (Katonah, New York, Blue Bridge, 2008.)

Dayle A. Friedman, *Jewish Visions for Aging. A Professional Guide for Fostering Wholeness. Text and Tradition. Aging and Meaning. Family*

---

210   Craig Kennet Miller, Address given at Boomerstock, Nashville, TN, sponsored by the United Methodist Church, September 28 to October 1, 2016.

Caregiving. Livui Ruchani: Spiritual Accompaniment in Aging. Aging and Community. (Woodstock, Vermont, Jewish Lights Publishing, 2008.)

Harold G. Koenig, *Aging and God. Aging and God: spiritual pathways to mental health in midlife and later years.* (New York, Haworth Pastoral Press, 1994.)

Jeff Levin, *God, Faith, and Health: Exploring the Spirituality – Healing Connection.* (New York, John Wiley & Sons, 2001.)

Craig Kennet Miller, *Boomer Spirituality. Seven Values for the Second Half of Life.* (Nashville, Discipleship Ministries, The United Methodist Church, 2017).

Swinton, John, *Resurrecting the Person. Friendship and the Care of People with Mental Health Problems.* (Nashville, Abingdon Press, 2000.)

Tindal, Mardi. *Soul Maps. A Guide to the Mid-life Spirit.* (Toronto, United Church Publishing House, 2000.)

For Viewing

Away from Her, Sarah Polley, director, 2007.

Still Alice, Richard Glatzer, Wash Westmoreland, directors, 2015.

Re-Designing Your Life: A Practical Spirituality for the Second Half of Life, Sheila Macdonald Macgregor, Wib Dawson, videographer and editor, 2017.

Questions for Discussion

Watch Session Six of the videos that have been made to accompany this book and then discuss the following. Note: if you are leading a study group, you may not have time to discuss all the questions. Choose those that you feel will be most helpful to your group.

1. Read Genesis 1:27 and I Corinthians 6:19. According to scripture, there is a reason we should take care of our bodies, one that goes far beyond the current youth craze and glorification of beauty for beauty's sake. Why does the bible place emphasis on caring for our physical bodies?

2. Do you find the literature connecting better health and well-being with religious faith compelling? Why or why not?

3. Read Ephesians 6:11. How is hope an integral part of good health?

4. Read John 15:15. How does Jesus look upon us and what difference should this make in our lives and especially in our relationship with God?

5. Read Luke 19:1–10 and John 4:1–26. What do we learn about the nature of the friendship Jesus offered to others? Consider Jesus's friendships also with the disciples, with Mary, Martha, and Lazarus, and with the beloved disciple. What do we learn about what it means to share in the ministry of friendship? What do you do if your offer of friendship or attempt to reach out is rejected or met with hostility? How can we begin to place less emphasis on "fixing" people and instead lift up the ministry of accompaniment and friendship in our own time?

6. Recall a time when someone really listened to your thoughts. What was this like for you?

7. In his book, *Aging Matters*, Stevens quotes James Houston and Michael Parker: "caregiving will be the great test of character this century" (Stevens, p. 109). Do you agree? Why? Read the fifth commandment in Exodus 20:12. Read also Ephesians 6:2. How do we honour and care for our elderly loved ones without detriment to our own health and well-being? Is there a limit to what our elderly loved ones or adult children can ask of us? If we are caregivers, how do we find spiritual nourishment and strength as we undertake this important ministry? How can the church provide help to those who are called to be caregivers?

8. How can the telling of our stories help both the one being cared for and the caregiver?

9. How does the practice of gratitude help us to let go of those we need to leave behind and cherish what we have? If you have been keeping a gratitude journal since session one, talk about how this exercise has been helpful to you.

10. (a) Visit Rabbi Richard Address's website: jewishsacredaging. com Read through the examples of religious rituals he has posted to his site and discuss. (b) Think back to a time in your life when a simple meal or event took on a sacramental nature. What was it about this event that made it so special? Try creating a ritual for a milestone you are facing in the second half of your life. Share it with some close friends or others in your study group. Have fun!

Chapter 7:
Inviting the Neighbours Over

A New Beginning: Retiring to, Not from Something

In a previous chapter, we talked about those things we need to leave behind, as well as some of the things we want to keep. We also began to talk about creating a legacy through the writing of an ethical will. In this chapter, we continue our discussion about creating a legacy. We also consider what it means to see ourselves not as people who are "retiring *from*" something, but rather as those who are "retiring *to*" something. As we complete our transition, we celebrate a new beginning.

Let's return to our metaphor of the house. Now that we have finished our renovations, kept what we think we'll need in our refurbished space, discarded what doesn't serve us anymore, and moved in, there is one thing we still need to do. We need to invite the neighbours over! And who are our neighbours? According to Jesus's Parable of the Good Samaritan in Luke 10:25–37, our neighbours are those who need our love and compassion. In short, our neighbour is everyone we encounter in life.

At Siloam United Church, where I have served for ten years, we have a contemporary building that has many big, bright picture windows. Sometimes, the light in the sanctuary is so intense that people actually wear their sunglasses during worship! Al Appleby, who was on the building committee when the new building was erected in 1988, says that the big windows are no accident. They aren't just about letting lots of natural light into the building, although that, too, is important. Their primary purpose, says Al, is to beckon our people out into the neighbourhood to serve God's world. Just as a real home does not stop at the edge of a well-manicured lawn, so, too, should a church extend its love to those outside its doors and beyond the parameters of its property, especially to those in need. Seeking to remain faithful to the mandate given us by Jesus, we invite others in, while at the same time going out to where they live. Likewise, the house that is our life must include space (and time) for others. The love we share in our home must move us beyond the walls we have constructed to attend to the needs of the wider community. We have inherited a wonderful treasure in the faith that has been passed down to us by previous generations, and now we have become its custodians. As stewards of this treasure, we must remember, however, that it has been given to us for one purpose only—so that we may share it with others.

Trivialized Existence Versus a Life of Service to Neighbour

One of the dangers we discussed at the outset of our study was the temptation to let others decide how we will spend these extra years with which we have been blessed, what Bateson calls the atrium of our life. Will we be proactive or reactive? As Christensen says, we can live our lives "by default, or we can live these years by design."[211] The choice is ours.

---

211   Janet Christensen Interview, July 2016.

Television and magazine commercials aimed at those in life's second half constantly feature older people having the time of their lives, travelling all over North America in their RVs, golfing, cycling, walking along beautiful sandy beaches, or dining at posh restaurants. Some even depict them engaging in death-defying sports like bungee jumping or skydiving. The message is that life at this stage should be fun and exciting. After all, we've earned it! Instead of inviting us into the abundant life promised by Jesus to all who would take up their cross and follow him, these ads promise 24/7 recreation and a life in which we no longer need to worry about making a difference in our community. However, those who only focus on having fun soon discover that it is not fun at all, but instead often leads to feelings of emptiness and depression. What is the answer? A life of service.

A Life of Service

The brilliant Jewish theologian Abraham Joshua Heschel taught that too much emphasis on leisure and relaxation leads to "the trivialization of existence."[212] It's like trying to be happy. When you aim for happiness, you are sure to miss it every time, but focus instead on helping and living for others, and you will be happy beyond your wildest dreams. Recall Schweitzer's words, again, when addressing a group of university students: "The only ones of you who will ever be truly happy are those of you who seek and find a way to serve." Or as Jesus said, "For those who want to save their life will lose it, and those who lose their life for my sake will find it." (Matthew 16:25)

---

212   Abraham Joshua Heschel, "To Grow in Wisdom," in *The Insecurity of Freedom.* (Philadelphia: Jewish Publication Society, 1966), 70-84.

As we have already noted, many of the great heroes of the Old Testament received their call from God at an advanced age. Abraham was seventy-five, and his wife Sarah was also elderly when they left their home and all that they had grown to love there to set off for the land God promised them (Genesis 12:1). Then there was Moses, who was eighty when he left his father-in-law's employ and took up the call to lead God's people out of slavery in Egypt. There was Naomi, who also made a long and treacherous journey back to her homeland with her daughter-in-law Ruth. Having lost everything—her youthfulness, her husband, and her two sons—she nevertheless carried on because of her own sense of responsibility for the future. Indeed, because of Naomi, the widowed Ruth found a new husband and gave birth to a son who ensured the continuation of her late husband's family line. Largely because of Naomi's resilience, the family's legacy was secured. These people chose to take the wisdom they had accrued through many years of experience in the school of life and place it in God's hands. They responded to God's call to embark, not on a life of amusement and frivolity, but, rather, on one fraught with hardship and danger, yet also filled with deep meaning and purpose. And that made all the difference.

Sadly, the life of service and sacrifice epitomized by the great heroes of the bible runs counter to our expectations for retirement today. Instead, what Stevens has called "institutionalized sloth" is now the norm.[213] Stevens believes that men and women should keep on working, if possible, until life's end. He notes that nowhere in the scriptures will you find the notion of retirement or "Freedom 55." In fact, in the opening pages of the bible, the mandate to work is intimately related to our

---

213   Stevens, *Work Matters*, 15.

identity as the image of God (Genesis 1:26). Moreover, as Christensen notes, it is not unusual for people, especially men, to suffer a heart attack or even die within the first six months of retirement.[214] I truly believe, for example, that the only thing that saved my father was that he could keep his law practice open, at least part-time, until well past his eightieth year.

But dying with one's boots on may not be an option for everyone and, indeed, those of us with good pensions need to ask ourselves if it does not also border on the unconscionable. A friend of mine who is a fitness instructor shared with me recently how one of her regular clients, a retired teacher, told her that she would have to miss the next few weeks of aerobic classes because she needed to go back and do some supply teaching for a month or so. Then she smiled brightly at my friend and exclaimed that she was planning a six-week vacation in Europe and she just needed a month or two of supply teaching, and she would have her holiday paid for! My friend groaned inwardly. She has two well-qualified and eager-to-work young adult children who are unable to secure full-time employment.

This is not to say that there are not many people who need to work well beyond retirement age to make ends meet. And it's not to say that people who provide a service should not receive some financial

---

214   Craig Kennet Miller, *Boomer Spirituality. Seven Values for the Second Half of Life*, pp. 47-48. Commenting on the suicide of comedian and actor Robin Williams in 2014, Miller writes that "Boomer men are sixty percent more likely to kill themselves than men in their parents' or grandparents' generations." Miller notes that factors contributing to the increase of loneliness in these second-half-of-life men include the increased divorce rate among boomer men, the loss of jobs during the Great Recession of 2008, and a lack of connection to a faith community that can support them.

remuneration. As the saying goes, the labourer is worthy of his or her hire. It's simply to note that this is a very complicated issue and one that may become more challenging as the years pass. On the other hand, it can be argued that, as men and women live longer, we need people to work longer to help carry the burden of paying for health care and government pensions.

Perhaps the major point to take away here is that work is an essential part of who we are as human beings who have been made in God's image. For those who can do so, volunteer work can be very satisfying personally and also serve the needs of the wider community. We do not always need to be paid for what we do, especially if we are fortunate enough to have the resources that enable us to give our toil freely and generously. But if we are to retain our humanity and fulfill our God-given calling, we do need to do some work. With so many gifts and talents, and with wisdom garnered from valuable experience in the workforce or the school of life, we have an obligation to serve God and our fellow human beings. This obligation is highlighted in an address Rabbi Heschel gave fifty-seven years ago to the 1961 White House Conference on Aging:

> What a person lives by is not only a sense of belonging, but a sense of indebtedness. The need to be needed corresponds to a fact: something is asked of a man, of every man. Advancing in years must not be taken to mean a process of suspending the requirements and commitments under which a person lives. To be is to obey. A person must never cease to be.[215]

---

215   Heschel, "To Grow in Wisdom," 70–84.

Mitzvot

Heschel's words are both profound and true. The Jewish tradition in which he was reared, as was our Lord, has much to teach us. One of these traditions, which can be particularly helpful to us as we enter the second half of life, is highlighted by Friedman in her work on Jewish wisdom for the aging. This is the Jewish concept of *mitzvot*. The simple meaning of this word is "command" or "divine commandment." Many of us are familiar with the Jewish coming of age ritual *bar mitzvah* or *bat mitzvah*, which means "son of the commandment" or "daughter of the commandment." In common usage, a *mitzvah* means a good deed, as in "Go and do a mitzvah and help Mrs. Green with her groceries."

Friedman sees these divine commandments more "as invitations to holiness."[216] They are opportunities to live out the covenant that God forged with God's people on Mount Sinai, to which every Jew since has been bound. It is through the practice of *mitzvot* that one remains faithful to God and finds meaning and purpose in life. Like Heschel, Friedman believes that everyone is obligated to the *mitzvot*, regardless of their age:

> This potential for meaning has no end point. There is no retirement from a life of *mitzvot* nor any senior citizen discount. We are called to hallow our lives every day for as long as we live. In this understanding, as we grow older, we are as bound to *mitzvot* as any other adult. We sense that something is expected of us, that our actions matter, that we can transcend recreation and emptiness. This is a refreshingly different message

---

216   Friedman, *Jewish Wisdom for Growing Older,* 115.

from the ones transmitted by our contemporary culture. We are always connected, always called, to hear and respond to the call of the mitzvah.[217]

Friedman notes that while the call of *mitzvah* is for life, the obligation is to fulfill this duty only as one is able. If one becomes limited by illness, for example, the expectations are adjusted accordingly. As she notes, this is made expressly clear in the *Book of Deuteronomy*, which recounts God's command to the Israelites. Here, I use the version that Peterson provides in *The Message*:

> This commandment that I'm commanding you today isn't too much for you, it's not out of your reach. It's not on a high mountain—you don't have to get mountaineers to climb the peak and bring it down to your level and explain it before you can live it. And it's not across the ocean—you don't have to send sailors out to get it, bring it back, and then explain it before you can live it. No. The word is right here and now—as near as the tongue in your mouth, as near as the heart in your chest. Just do it! (Deuteronomy 30:11–14).[218]

In other words, God never demands more of us than we can do. But—and here's the clincher—God still expects us to be faithful and accountable, at least to the best of our ability. As Stanley Hauerwas puts it in his wonderful book, *Growing Old in Christ,* for people of faith, "there is no 'Florida'—even if they happen to live in Florida.

---

217   Ibid., 116.

218   *The Message. The Bible in Contemporary Language.* Eugene H. Petersen, translator. (Carol Stream, Illinois, NavPress, 2014).

That is, we must continue to be present to those who have made us what we are so that we can make future generations what they are called to be."[219] In speaking about our call as Christians, he adds that our aging "cannot be a lost opportunity." It cannot be cashed in for a lifetime pass to Disney World. In short, Christians do not retire. Like Jews, we are called to serve God our whole life long.

While Jews regard the law given on Mount Sinai as the basis of the covenant that binds them to God, Christians believe that baptism is God's signature and seal on God's covenant of grace. Baptism is given to us by God as the pledge of God's love and faithfulness, but both the Creator and the created have their parts to play in baptism. While God's part always comes first, we are nevertheless expected to play our part by answering God's call, by keeping the faith, and by following in the way of Jesus. As our United Church *Song of Faith* states, "Baptism signifies the nurturing, sustaining, and transforming power of God's love and our grateful response to that grace."[220] The way we live out the promises of the covenant of baptism is by responding to God's grace and engaging in a life of service. In other words, we reach out to our neighbours with love and compassion.

Thankfulness

The reason we do this—the reason Jews practise *mitzvot*—is not to earn favour with God, but to thank God for the blessings of life. To quote again from our United Church *Song of Faith*, "Grateful for God's loving action, we cannot keep from singing." Studies now show

---

219   Stanley Hauerwas, *Growing Old in Christ* (Grand Rapids: Eerdmans, 2003), 182.

220   The United Church of Canada, *Song of Faith*.

that people who keep a regular gratitude journal are healthier, both physically and mentally.[221] The practice of giving thanks is important for people of every generation, but now, in the second half of life, it is essential to our health and well-being. With more years behind us than before us, with more aching joints than we knew we even had, and with the loss of family members and friends, we now understand that life cannot be taken for granted. Little wonder, then, that gratitude is a focus of nearly every great religion. It is also, as Beattie-Stokes writes, one of the chief signs that we have reached a point of spiritual maturity:

> Gratitude awakens us to beauty, to wonder, to love, to
> ourselves, and to others. Gratitude frees us to love and
> accept self and others; it enables us to discover our soul
> gifts and to give them away as the only fitting response
> to the Giver. Gratitude awakens a wise heart.[222]

It is gratitude that enables us to live the life of *mitzvot* and serve God and neighbour with love and faithfulness, even in challenging and difficult circumstances. It is gratitude that empowers us to live out our holy covenant with the God of Sinai and the promises of our baptism in Jesus Christ.

Creating a Mission Statement for the Second Half of Life

If gratitude moves us to desire a life of service, a personal mission statement helps us determine how and where we can best serve. Most businesses and organizations have a mission statement. However, long before the commercial world talked about mission, this term was used solely in connection with the Christian faith. The church had a

---

221   Ibid.

222   Beattie-Stokes, *A Heart of Wisdom*, 99.

mission. That mission was to "go therefore and make disciples of all nations." (Matthew 28:19) Jesus himself had a personal mission. He came, as he said, "that my joy may be in you and so that your joy may be complete." (John 15:11) At Siloam United Church, our mission statement is emblazoned above the entrance to our sanctuary, included in our weekly bulletins, and repeated every Sunday in our commissioning and benediction: "To be Christ to each other and God's world."

Sadly, most individuals do not have a mission statement. A lot of us have been content to "leave things to the snake." But a mission statement can provide us with clarity to enable us to be focused on what really matters to us, and then we can intentionally let other things go. Planning makes the difference between having a midlife crisis; a deadly boring second half; or a second half that is filled with meaning, service, and deep satisfaction. And far from being a straitjacket, having this kind of awareness about ourselves helps us to stay connected to the Spirit, which "blows where it chooses…So it is with everyone who is born of the Spirit." (John 3:8)

At this stage of life, we have a wealth of knowledge about ourselves that we did not have, for example, when we were graduating from high school or even university or our first apprenticeship. We have an idea of what we are passionate about, what our strengths are and where we perform best, how we interact with people, and how we react to varying situations. We also have a sense of how much "alone" time we need versus interaction with others, and we know whether we function better in a structured environment or one that is unstructured. We have completed our social portfolio and maybe have even written an ethical will. Now it's time to write a personal mission statement.

How to Write Your Personal Mission Statement

Step One:

Think about what makes you most passionate. What has made you angry or sad in the past? What articles in the newspaper or on the internet make you want to get up and do something? What painful experiences in your past could provide a passion for the future? Or think about something you are curious about. Just get something down, and begin there, rather than trying to get it right on the first try.

> - What causes, issues, and groups of people concern you most?

> - What change do you most want to help bring about in the world or right in your own neighbourhood?

Step Two:

Look back at the exercise you completed on strengths in chapter 5. Write down your three greatest strengths. (In the church, we refer to these as our *spiritual gifts*.) What strengths can you build on? Identifying and building on your strengths is going to be a major factor in your successful transition to the second half of life.

Share your findings with a trusted friend who knows you well. Listen to your friend's feedback and rewrite if you need to do so.

Step Three:

Develop your personal mission statement. Keep this in a place where you are likely to see it every day. For example, you may paste it to the bathroom mirror or the refrigerator.

According to management guru Peter Drucker, a mission statement is designed to say what we do, why we do it, and what we want to be remembered for. It is not intended to describe how we will go about doing what we do because our methods and tactics will change as our environment and technology change. It is important to be flexible, while keeping one's focus on the mission. Many industries have suffered because they lost sight of their true mission. For example, the Swiss thought their mission was to produce fine mechanical watches. They lost sight of the fact that their real mission was to help people tell time, and thus they lost a major market to the Japanese, who invented digital watches to help people tell time. Likewise, the train industry thought they were in the business of creating better and faster trains, when they were really in the transportation business. Hence, they missed an important opportunity to invest in air travel. Keep focussed on your mission and open to ever-new ways to share it!

Key elements in our personal mission statement:

- What is your greatest strength or area of competence?

- What kind of people or things do you care about the most?

- What difference do you dream you could make for those people or that cause?

What is your mission statement (calling)? Take a few minutes to fill in the blanks in the sentence below by inserting your top strengths, then the area of your passion based on what you know now, and then insert the kind of difference you most desire to make as a result.

My Strengths/Gifts:

My Passions:

The Impact I Want to Make:

SAMPLE MISSION STATEMENT:

With God's help I plan to use OR I am trusting God to use my _____(gifts/strengths) to serve_____(my area of passion), in order to _____(the impact or difference you want to make).

Stories to Accompany Us as We Settle into our Newly Renovated House . . .

First Nations author Velma Wallis tells a beautiful story to accompany us as we move into the second half of life.

> The tale opens with the people starving and desperate. The chief and the council decide to leave the two frail old women behind. It is thought they will only be a burden on the already suffering tribe.

> Bereft, the two old women can hardly believe that they have been left to fend on their own. However, they refuse to give in to their fate and soon set off to find a place at which they had camped many, many years earlier. It was a place that was both beautiful and fruitful. After six days of constant walking, tired and worn out, the women finally arrive at the camp.

The two old women survive the winter, and in the spring, they begin to prepare for the future in earnest. They trap muskrats, beavers, and rabbits. They smoke the meat to preserve it and make clothing and hats out of the skins of the animals. They catch great quantities of fish to preserve. They also gather firewood and stack it all around their camp for fuel for the winter.

Meanwhile, the rest of the tribe has suffered terribly. Several of their tribe have died from malnutrition, including some children. Barely surviving, those who remain decide to return to the camp.

When, eventually, they come upon the two old women, they are amazed to learn how well the women have managed without them. The women have plenty to eat and good furs to keep them warm. At this, the chief and the rest of the tribe realise their terrible mistake in sending the women away, for the old women have great wisdom to share. They can tell the others about places they visited when they were young. They know where to go in times of famine and hardship. They know how to survive in times of great difficulty. They therefore have much of value to teach the younger generations.

The chief and the tribe repent of their ways, and the old women give them clothing and share with them the food they have hunted and preserved. Most of all, they share their wisdom.[223]

We are the Meaning Keepers

Like the chief and his council in Wallis's story, our Western society has tended to undervalue those in the second half of life. To a large degree, in the words of Richard Rohr, we are "a first-half-of-life culture," focused mostly on the tasks we associate with the first half of life: establishing an identity, a home, relationships, friends, career, and security. Our institutions, including our churches, tend to encourage, support, reward, and validate these first-half-of-life tasks. Mired in what he calls the egocentric first stage of life, Rohr quotes Bill Plotkin, who says that we live in a "patho-adolescent culture."[224]

But a society that forgets those in the second half of life denies itself many important resources, as we see in this story of the two old women. Every society needs to have living exemplars or models who can serve as life's guides and replenish and nourish the rest of society. Every society needs its mentors, its "meaning and memory keepers," or what the Apostle Paul calls the "stewards of God's mysteries." (I Corinthians. 4:1) In other words, every society needs mature men and women who can show others the way.

Regrettably, even in cultures that have traditionally valued those who hold the sacred meanings of life and death, we are seeing an erosion of community values. Years ago, while interviewing many of the Elders of

---

223   Velma Wallis, *Two Old Women: An Alaska Legend of Betrayal, Courage and Survival* (New York: Harper Perennial, 1994). See also Clayton, *Called for Life*, 78-79.

224   Rohr, *Healing Our Violence*, 27.

the Anishinawbeg First Nation, my cousin Craig observed: "I talked to the oldest people I could find and the younger people had trouble listening because the elders were talking about places they had never been."[225] Because of the aggressive policy of assimilation, many of the young scorned their own traditions and abandoned the old ways.

Understandably, Rev. Matthew Stevens, an Elder in the Aamjiwnaang First Nation, deeply laments this development. In a recent conversation, I shared with Matthew that my sense is that First Nations peoples have always had a much greater respect for people in the second half of life and the wisdom and experience they bring to the life of the community. This is how Matthew responded to my comment:

> I think that's true as a broad generalization, but it is
> not necessarily so to the same degree with the younger
> generations as it was when I was growing up, and
> into my adulthood. The veneration of eldership is a
> phenomenon that, almost without exception, is true
> of every non-literate society, virtually anywhere in the
> world. When there is no physical means of recording
> and preserving the history and accumulated wisdom
> of a society, those who are specifically acknowledged
> and trained as the "wisdom keepers" are crucial to the
> community as a whole. "Book-learning" frequently
> serves to undermine that centrality by creating the
> illusion that genuine wisdom and accurate history can
> somehow be objectively written down, as opposed to
> being preserved in their appropriate context. There is

---

225   Conversation with Craig Macdonald, August 18, 2016, and Jenish, "Mapman of Temagami."

of course, no such thing as "objective history," for it is always written down by the victor; and the moment you place wisdom into the category of "book-learning," you rob it of the contextualization and mentoring function that makes it relevant. The result is a rationalization for past travesties, and trivialized drivel only suitable for Coutts-Hallmark inspirational cards and clever Facebook posts. It's quite possible that you'll be witnessing the passing of practical eldership.[226]

I pray that Matthew is wrong. I know he does, too. More than anything else, our world today needs elders who can bring the wisdom they've gleaned over a lifetime to the many pressing and life-threatening issues facing our planet. Both Bateson and University of Waterloo psychology professor, Igor Grossman, argue that those in the second half of life bring a special ability to look at issues from a much-needed "third-person perspective"[227] and hence are able to restore a sense of calm and "a dimension of long-term thinking to society."[228] These are gifts we cannot afford to ignore. With the enormity of the global problems we face, the wisdom, experience, and passion of our elders are needed now more than ever. We who find ourselves in the second half of life are thus in a unique position to make a difference in our houses of faith and our communities. We have an opportunity to lead the way, and to live out Christ's mission to the world he so loves.

---

226   Matthew Stevens email.
227   Paul Knowles, "Older and Wiser," *The United Church Observer,* July/August 2014, 16-17. Bateson, *Composing a Further Life,* 20.
228   Ibid.

The Witness of Simeon and Anna: Sentinels for the Messiah and "Meaning Keepers" Par Excellence

The scriptures call to us from across the ages with stories about people in the second half of life who have shared their wisdom and passion generously and taught us important life lessons. First, there is the story of the old prophet called Simeon:

> [21] And when eight days had passed, before His circumcision, His name was then called Jesus, the name given by the angel before He was conceived in the womb.
>
> [22] And when the days for their purification according to the law of Moses were completed, they brought Him up to Jerusalem to present Him to the Lord [23] (as it is written in the Law of the Lord, "Every firstborn male that opens the womb shall be called holy to the Lord"), [24] and to offer a sacrifice according to what was said in the Law of the Lord, "A pair of turtledoves or two young pigeons."
>
> [25] And there was a man in Jerusalem whose name was Simeon; and this man was righteous and devout, looking for the consolation of Israel; and the Holy Spirit was upon him. [26] And it had been revealed to him by the Holy Spirit that he would not see death before he had seen the Lord's Christ. [27] And he came in the Spirit into the temple; and when the parents brought in the child Jesus, to carry out for Him the custom of the Law, [28] then he took Him into his arms, and blessed God, and said,

²⁹ "Now Lord, You are releasing Your bond-servant to depart in peace,

According to Your word;

³⁰ For my eyes have seen Your salvation,

³¹ Which You have prepared in the presence of all peoples,

³² A light of revelation to the Gentiles,

And the glory of Your people Israel."

³³ And His father and mother were amazed at the things which were being said about Him. ³⁴ And Simeon blessed them and said to Mary His mother, "Behold, this Child is appointed for the fall and rise of many in Israel, and for a sign to be opposed— ³⁵ and a sword will pierce even your own soul—to the end that thoughts from many hearts may be revealed." (Luke 2:21–35 NASB.)

The words from Milton's sonnet come to mind as we reflect upon this wise elder: "They also serve who only stand and wait."[229] Simeon has waited faithfully and over many decades to be a witness to the coming of the Messiah. Now his dream has been fulfilled, and he can die in peace. Simeon's job as a sentinel for the Messiah is done.

What would it mean for us to become like Simeon and serve as sentinels for the Messiah? Perhaps it's this. As we age, there is less need to be busy

---

229   John Milton, "When I Consider How My Light is Spent," 1674.

and productive and doing, and a greater call for us to be reflective and to consider all that has been and is. To use Vaillant's words, it is the sentinel's job to serve as the "keeper of meaning." But in preserving the best of our faith traditions and stories, the sentinel also stands in a place that allows him or her to provide the kind of helpful reflection and wise counsel that Grossman and Bateson argue is so badly needed in our time. The great spiritual writer Ronald Rolheiser says that, as we enter the second half of life, our discipleship must become one of reflection rather than productivity.[230]

In this case, the sentinel is also a "truth-teller." From his vantage point of having lived many decades, Simeon knows that Jesus's life will not be an easy one. Many will oppose him, plot against him, and ultimately betray and crucify him. Those who follow him must be prepared to die in the cause. His mother Mary will suffer profoundly because of this child she has borne. The kind of truth-telling that is required if one is to serve as a sentinel for Jesus need not be ruthless or unkind; but it does call for a sobering honesty and transparency that may be difficult for us to hear, as they must have been for Mary and Joseph.

Finally, as sentinels for the Messiah, we must ever keep before us Simeon's vision of the prophetic hope found in Isaiah 49:6, that Israel is to be a "light to the nations." The salvation brought by the Messiah's birth, Simeon announces, is for "all peoples." As Christ's sentinels, therefore, we must be vigilant on our watch against those who would attempt to erode or restrict God's graciousness. The love of God that we meet in Jesus Christ is for all people everywhere, including the differently-abled and regardless of colour or class, religion or creed, race or nationality, education or language,

---

230   Ronald Rolheiser, *Sacred Fire: A Vision for a Deeper Human and Christian Maturity* (New York: Image, 2014), 299.

gender or sexual orientation, friend or stranger, rich or poor, marital status or age. As sentinels for Jesus, our task is not to ensure that walls are kept secure and insurmountable, but rather to ensure the gates to God's love are constantly kept widely open and easily accessible to all and by all. For as Jesus proclaimed, "In my Father's house are many dwelling places" or rooms. (John 14:2) As Rolheiser points out, this is not a reference to the number of rooms in God's house. It's about the expanse or "scope of God's heart," which includes all people everywhere.[231] As we take up residence in our newly renovated home, we are called to practise this open-door policy and radical hospitality of our Lord.

The story of Anna the prophetess is another example of a biblical witness to the positive influence we can have in the second half of life. Her story below has much to teach us.

[36] There was also a prophet, Anna the daughter of Phanuel, of the tribe of Asher. She was of a great age, having lived with her husband seven years after her marriage, [37] then as a widow to the age of eighty-four. She never left the temple but worshiped there with fasting and prayer night and day. [38] At that moment she came, and began to praise God and to speak about the child to all who were looking for the redemption of Jerusalem. (Luke 2:36-38)

We discover quite a few facts about Anna in this scripture passage. She is in the second half of life. She is a widow. She worships, she fasts, and she prays. She gives thanks to God in all things. No doubt she has known great suffering in her life, having been widowed while still a very young woman. But she does not allow her suffering to harden her or cause her to become bitter or unforgiving or resentful. Instead,

---

231   Ibid., 271.

a profound sense of gratitude informs her very being, allowing her to live joyfully and faithfully. As we proclaim in the United Church *Song of Faith*, "Grateful for God's loving action, [Anna] cannot keep from singing." Her thankful and empathetic spirit flows out to others, whom she blesses by teaching them about the Messiah. We're told that she never leaves the Temple. I get the feeling that she leads a very engaged life—she may live at the Temple, but more likely, she is there when the doors open each day, and she does not leave until they close.

Reflection and Prayer

What would it mean for us to pray constantly, as Anna does? Does this mean that we should always be at full-time prayer? While Rollheiser believes that we should seize every opportunity to engage in both liturgical prayer (the formal prayers we pray in community or while we are in public worship) and the less formal, more personal, contemplative prayers we pray when alone, he sees the biblical injunction to "pray always" more as an invitation "to live our lives against a certain horizon."[232] He uses the example of the married person who goes on a business trip and is engaged in many meetings and workshops or networking events. While he or she may not have much time to speak with or even think about the partner or children who have been left back home, nevertheless it is the family that keeps him or her grounded, and that constitutes the most important relationship. Prayer is like that, says Rollheiser. It keeps us anchored to God. It is the backdrop against which all our thoughts and actions take place.

Some scholars have observed that there is an interesting change that takes place in the nature of our prayers as we enter the second half of

---

232   Ibid., 176-177.

life. Such is the finding of Robert C. Atchley, a specialist in the field of aging and spirituality. Atchley writes that, in his twenty-year study of adults in Anna's age bracket, he discovered a tendency to engage much more in contemplative prayer and meditation than petitionary prayer. He writes: "Petitionary prayer asks something of God. Meditative prayer has little form. The practitioner simply 'waits upon the Lord.' The point is to be present, open, attuned to messages from God, yet not expecting any specific experience."[233]

It is the latter, I think, that best describes the kind of prayer that defines Anna's life: meditative, contemplative, always open, and attuned to the voice of God's Spirit. Yet, as with all true spirituality, Anna's prayer life leads her to reach out to others in love and service. Think about it. Every day people come to the Temple to pray and offer their sacrifices. Can't you just see Anna welcoming and encouraging and teaching and advising the people who visit there? Can you not hear her speaking about her faith and the promised Messiah? Like old Simeon, she is acting as a mentor and witness to others. She is the "memory keeper," the one who keeps the stories alive by sharing them with all whom she meets. As such, she is a servant of Christ and a steward of the mysteries of God.

The stories of Simeon and Anna provide us with beautiful examples of how to live in the second half of life. They teach us about the importance of reflection and prayer, about the centrality of doing all things with a joyful and thankful heart, about honesty and truth-telling, about inclusivity and hospitality, and most of all about sharing the Good News of God's love in Jesus Christ with those who follow. As

---

233   Robert C. Atchley, *Spirituality and Aging* (Baltimore: Johns Hopkins University Press, 2009), 129.

we move into the house that will be our home in the second half of life, we can do no better than to take these ancient New Testament prophets as our models and mentors. May their example challenge and inspire us to seize the life Christ wants to give us that we may live fully and joyfully in the afternoon of life.

For Further Reading

Robert C. Atchley, *Spirituality and Aging*. (Baltimore, The Johns Hopkins University Press, 2009.)

Anne Beattie-Stokes, *A Heart of Wisdom. Inspiration and Instruction for Conscious Elderhood.* (North Charleston, SC, Booksurge Publishing, 2009.)

Dayle Friedman, *Jewish Wisdom for Growing Older. Finding Your Grit & Grace Beyond Midlife.* (Woodstock, Vermont, For People of All Faiths, All Backgrounds, Jewish Lights Publishing, 2015.)

Stanley Hauerwas, *Growing Old in Christ*. (Grand Rapids, Eerdmans, 2003.)

Ronald Rollheiser, *Sacred Fire. A Vision for a Deeper Human and Christian Maturity.* (New York, Image, 2014.)

Velma Wallis, *Two Old Women: An Alaska Legend of Betrayal, Courage, and Survival.* (New York, Harper Collins, 1993.)

For Viewing

Re-Designing Your Life: A Practical Spirituality for the Second Half of Life, Sheila Macdonald Macgregor, Wib Dawson, videographer and editor, 2017.

Questions for Discussion

Watch Session Seven of the videos that have been made to accompany this book and then discuss the following. Note: if you are leading a study group, you may not have time to discuss all the questions. Choose those that you feel will be most helpful to your group. Before you end your sessions together, be sure to take a few minutes to watch the closing video.

1. Abraham Joshua Heschel wrote that too much emphasis on leisure and relaxation leads to "the trivialization of existence." Do you think the retirement industry promotes the trivialization of which Heschel wrote years ago? How? Why is it necessary for us to bring a faith perspective to our retirement years?

2. Do you agree with Stevens that we should work until we die? Why or why not? Is "Freedom 55" an option for the person of faith? Consider this question in light of Paul's *Letter to the Galatians* 5:1, "For freedom Christ has set us free. Stand firm, then, and do not be subject again to the yoke of slavery." How does our freedom in Christ free us to serve Christ and his world?

3. Why is it important to practice the art of gratitude? How might you begin to make this a central spiritual practice in your own life? (If you have been keeping a Gratitude Journal, talk about how this has been helpful to you.)

4. What is the lesson we should take away from Velma Wallis's story about the two old women? Why should we share this with our children?

5. Matthew Stevens laments the demise of the elder in First Nations communities. How can we begin to train wisdom elders in our own community and why is this so important to the future of our world?

6. Re-read the stories of Simeon and Anna in the second chapter of Luke's Gospel. How can we learn from their examples and how do their stories provide us with much-needed models for living in the second half of life?

7. Dr. Janet Miller asks: "If someone were to do a Google search of your name, what would you like them to read about you?"[234]

8. Write a personal mission statement. Consider how your gifts and strengths can serve God's world.

---

234   Dr. Janet Miller, 7th International Conference on Ageing and Spirituality, Chicago, Illinois, June 4th – 7th, 2017.

Bibliography

Adams, Michael. *Sex in the Snow: The Surprising Revolution in Canadian Social Values.* (Toronto, Viking Canada, 1997.)

_____*Staying Alive. How Canadian Baby Boomers Will Work, Play and Find Meaning.* (Toronto, Viking Canada, 2010.)

Address, Richard F. "Exile and Love" in *Jewish Sacred Aging*, February 2, 2012.

_____, *Seekers of Meaning. Baby Boomers, Judaism, and the Pursuit of Healthy Aging.* (New York, URJ Press, 2012.)

Albert, Susan Wittig. *Writing from Life. Telling Your Soul's Story.* (New York, The Putnam Publishing Group, 1996.)

Atchley, Robert C., *Spirituality and Aging.* (Baltimore, The Johns Hopkins University Press, 2009.)

Baines, Barry K. *Ethical Wills. Putting Your Values on Paper.* (De Capo Press, 2002.)

Bali, Dr. Susan. "Five Steps to Finding Your Passion," *Psychology Today,* Posted May 8, 2012.

Bausch, William J., *A World of Stories for Preachers and Teachers.* (Mystic, CT, Twenty-Third Publications, 1998.)

_____, *60 More Seasonal Homilies.* (Mystic, CT, Twenty-Third Publications, 2002.)

Bateson, Mary Catherine, *Composing A Life.* (New York, Grove Press, 1989.)

_____, *Re-Composing A Life.* (New York, A Knopf e Book, 2010.)

Beattie-Stokes, Anne. *A Heart of Wisdom. Inspiration and Instruction for Conscious Elderhood.* (North Charleston, SC, Booksurge Publishing, 2009.)

Benke, William and Benke, Le Etta. *The Generation Driven Church: Evangelizing Boomers, Busters, and Millennials.* (Cleveland, OH: Pilgrim Press, 2002.)

Bianchi, Eugen C., *Aging as a Spiritual Journey.* (New York, Crossroad, 1990.)

Bibby, Reginald., *The Boomer Factor. What Canada's Most Famous Generation is Leaving Behind.* (B.C., Wood Lake Publishing, 2006.)

Bieble, David E. and Koenig, Harold C. *New Light on Depression. Help, Hope and Answers for the Depressed and Those Who Love Them.* (Grand Rapids, Zondervan, 2004.)

Boone, Fran. Interview with author. December 2, 2016.

Bowen, Kurt. *Christians in a Secular World. The Canadian Experience.* (Montreal, McGill-Queen's University Press; 2005.)

Brack, Tara. *"Growing Up Unworthy,"* blog, April 19, 2013.

Bridges, William. *Embracing Life's Most Difficult Moments.* (Cambridge, DaCapo Press, 2001.)

_____, *The Way of Transition.* (Cambridge, Da Capo Press, 2001.)

_____ *Transitions: Making Sense of Life's Changes,* 2nd edition. (Cambridge, DaCapo Press, 2004.)

Buechner, Frederick. *Beyond Words: Daily Readings in the ABCs of Faith.* (San Francisco, Harper, 2004.)

_____, *Wishful Thinking: A Seeker's ABC.* (New York, Harper One, 1993.)

Butler-Bass, Diana. *Christianity After Religion: The End of Church and the Birth of a New Spiritual Awakening.* (New York, Harper One, 2012.)

Butt, Bill and Butt, Karen. Interview with author, October 21, 2016.

Carstensen, Laura. *A Long Bright Future.* (New York, Public Affairs, 2011.)

_____, "Baby Boomers Are Isolating Themselves as They Age," *Time,* May 12, 2016.

Chan, Cindy. "Stress of Caregiving Hurts Baby Boomers," *Epoch Times,* June 8, 2010.

Chatterton, Ryan. "The Ultimate Secret to Discovering Your Passion". *The Huffington Post,* April 9, 2013.

Chittister, Joan. *The Gift of Years. Growing Old Gracefully.* (Katonah, New York, Blue Bridge, 2008.)

Christensen, Janet. Interview with author, July 19, 2016, London, Ont.

Christensen, Janet. "It's Not Just About Money!" in Eastman, Linda Ellis, editor. *Secrets for Life After 50!* (Prospect, Kentucky, Professional Woman Publishing, 2014), pp. 81-91.

Clayton, Paul C. *Called for Life. Finding Meaning in Retirement.* (Herndon Virginia, The Alban Institute, 2008.)

Clements, William M. and Koenig, Harold G. *Aging and God: Spiritual Pathways to Mental Healthy in Midlife and Later years.* (London, Routledge, 1994.)

Cox, Harvey. *On Not Leaving It to the Snake.* (New York, MacMillan, 1967.)

Cohen, Gene D. *The Creative Age. Awakening Human Potential in the Second Half of Life.* (New York, Quill, 2000.)

Daniel, Lillian. *When "Spiritual but Not Religious" Is Not Enough. Seeing God in Surprising Places, Even the Church.* (New York, Jericho Books, 2013.)

De Bono, Norman. "Canadians 65 and older have highest suicide rate of any group in the country," *The London Free Press*, Sunday, June 16, 2013.

Dennis, Wendy. "How Grey Divorce Became the New Normal," *Zoomer Magazine*, June 3, 2016.

De St. Aubin, Ed, McAdams, Dan. P., Kim, Tae-Chang. *The Generative Society. Caring for Future Generations.* (Washington, DC, American Psychological Association, 2004.)

Eastman, Linda Ellis, editor. *Secrets for Life After 50!* (Prospect, Kentucky, Professional Woman Publishing, 2014.)

Elliott, Trisha, "The Gratitude Effect," *The United Church of Canada Observer,* October 2016.

Erikson, Erik H. *Childhood and Society.* (New York, W. W. Norton & Company, 1985 Kindle edition.)

_____, *The Life Cycle Completed.* Extended Version with New Chapters on the Ninth Stage of Development by Joan M. Erikson. (New York, W. W. Norton & Company, Kindle edition.)

Freed, Rachel. *Women's Lives. Passing Your Beliefs and Blessing to Future Generations. Creating Your Own Spiritual-Ethical Will.* (Minneapolis, Fairview Press, 2003.)

Friedman, Dayle A. *Jewish Visions for Aging. A Professional Guide for Fostering Wholeness. Text and Tradition. Aging and Meaning. Family Caregiving. Livui Ruchani: Spiritual Accompaniment in Aging. Aging and Community.* (Woodstock, Vermont, Jewish Lights Publishing, 2008.)

_____, *Jewish Wisdom for Growing Older. Finding Your Grit & Grace Beyond Midlife.* (Woodstock, Vermont, For People of All Faiths, All Backgrounds, Jewish Lights Publishing, 2015.)

Foot, David K. Boom, *Bust & Echo. How to profit from the coming demographic shift.* (Toronto, Macfarlane, Walter & Ross, 1996.)

Freedman, Marc. *Prime Time. How Baby Boomers Will Revolutionize Retirement and Transform America.* (New York, BBS Public Affairs, 1999.)

Galbraith, Susan. Conversation with author, September 4, 2016.

Girard, Lisa. "How to Find Your Passion in Five Creativity Exercises," *Entrepreneur.*

Goff, James R. Jr. "The Faith That Claims," *Christianity Today*, 34. (February 1990.)

Haemmelmann, Keith A. *Growing Older, Thinking Younger: Ministry with Boomers.* (Cleveland, The Pilgrim Press, 2012.)

Hall, Douglas John. *Bound and Free. A Theologian's Journey.* (Minneapolis, Fortress Press, 2005.)

_____ *"Stewards of the Mysteries of God,"* lecture at Lutheran Theological Seminary at Gettysburg Seminary on October 27, 2005. The talk was sponsored by the Stewardship of Life Institute and the Arthur Larson Stewardship Council. Copyright © 2005 Douglas John Hall.

_____*Waiting for Gospel. An Appeal to the Dispirited Remnants of Protestant Establishment.* (Eugene, Oregon, Cascade Books, 2012.)

_____*What Christianity is Not. An Exercise in "Negative" Theology.* (Eugene, Oregon, Cascade Books, 2013.)

_____, *"Stewardship as a Human Vocation,"* Stewardship of Life, September 7, 2010. 2010 Stewardship of Life Institute, 61 Seminary Ridge, Gettysburg, PA 17325

Hansen, R. Jack and Haas, Jerry P. *Retirement as Spiritual Pilgrimage: Stories, Scripture & Practices for the Journey.* (Create Space Independent Publishing, 2015.)

Hanson, Amy. *Baby Boomers and Beyond: Tapping the Ministry Talents and Passions of Adults over 50.* (San Francisco, Jossey-Bass Leadership Network Series, #45, 2010)

Hauerwas, Stanley, *Growing Old in Christ.* (Grand Rapids, Eerdmans, 2003.)

Hassler, Christine. Blog, November 29, 2012.

Heschel, Abraham Joshua, "To Grow in Wisdom," *The Insecurity of Freedom.* (Philadelphia, Jewish Publication Society, 1960), pp. 70-81.

Hodges, Glenn. "'The Big Shift,' Interview with Marc Freedman on Midlife Crisis," AARP Bulletin, May 12, 2011.

_____, *Shaping A Life of Significance for Retirement.* (Nashville, Upper Room Books, 2010.)

Hoge, Dean R., Benton Johnson, and Donald A. Luidens. *Vanishing boundaries: the religion of mainline Protestant baby boomers.* (Louisville, KY: Westminster/John Knox Press, 1994.)

Jenish, D'Arcy, "Mapman of Temagami," *Legion Canada's Military History Magazine*, May 1, 2006.

Johnson, Richard P. "Shaping a New Vision of Faith Formation for maturing Adults: Sixteen Fundamental Task," Lifelong Faith, Spring, 2007.

Jung, Carl. *Modern Man in Search of a Soul.* (New York, Harcourt, Brace and World, 1933.)

Kadelkova, "Relationships: Understanding the risky sex habits of Canadian baby boomers." *Canadian Living Magazine*, December 3, 2010.

King, Romansana. "The ultimate home maintenance guide. A complete schedule of when to do what . . . and how much it costs." *Money Sense*, October 6, 2011.

Knowles, Paul, "Older and Wiser," *The United Church Observer*. July/August 2014, pp. 16-17.

Koenig, Harold G. *Aging and God. Aging and God: spiritual pathways to mental health in midlife and later years.* (New York, Haworth Pastoral Press, 1994.)

Kornfield, Jack and Feldman, Christina, *Stories of the Spirit.* (San Francisco, Harper, 1991.)

Kotre, John N. *Outliving the Self. Generativity and the Interpretation of Lives.* (Baltimore, Maryland, John Hopkins Press, 1984.)

Lackey, Neil, and Lackey, Linda, Interview with author, September 16, 2016, Wellesley, Ont.

Laslett, Peter. *A Fresh Map of Life: The Emergence of the Third Age.* (Cambridge, Harvard University Press, 1991.)

Lawrence-Lightfoot, Sara, *The Third Chapter. Passion, Risk and Adventure in the 25 Years After 50.* (New York, Sarah Crichton Books, Farrar, Straus and Giroux, 2010.)

Levin, Jeff. *God, Faith, and Health: Exploring the Spirituality-Healing Connection.* (New York, John Wiley & Sons, 2001.)

Levinson, Daniel J. *The Seasons of a Man's Life.* (Toronto, Ballantine Books, 1978.)

_____with Judy D. Levinson. *The Seasons of a Woman's Life.* (New York. Ballantine Books. 1996.)

Link, Mark. *100 Stories for Special Occasion Homilies.* (Allen, Texas, Tabor Publishing, 1992.)

Macdonald, Craig. Conversation with author, August 18, 2016.

Macgregor, Sheila. "Bring Back the Baby Boomers", *The United Church Observer*, December 2016.

_____ "Capture Your Life Story", *Huron-Perth Boomers*, Fall, 2016.

_____ "How to Create Rituals for this Stage of Life", *Zoomer Magazine*, October 19th, 2017.

_____ "Interview with Jane Kuepfer", *The United Church Observer*, January 2018.

Mayo Clinic Staff, "Friendships: Enrich your life and improve your health. Discover the connection between health and friendship, and how to promote and maintain healthy friendships." June 9, 2011.

McClelland, David. *Human Motivation.* (Cambridge, Cambridge University Press, 1988.)

_____, "Human Motivation Theory," www.learnmanagement2.com/DavidMcClelland.htm

McIntosh, Gary L., *One Church, Four Generations: Understanding and Reaching All Ages in your Church.* (Baker Books, Grand Rapids, MI, 2007)

Mellinger, Dr. Marianne. Interview with author. Tuesday, July 26th, 2016, Conrad Grebel College, University of Waterloo, Waterloo, Ontario.

Mercadante, Linda A. *Belief without Borders. Inside the Minds of the Spiritual but not Religious.* (New York, Oxford University Press, 2014.)

Miller, Craig Kennet. Address given at *Boomerstock*, Nashville, Tennessee. Sponsored by the United Methodist Church, September 28 to October 1, 2016.

_____, *Baby Boomer Spirituality. Ten Essential Values of Generation.* (Nashville, Discipleship Resources, 1992.)

_____, *Boomer Spirituality. Seven Values for the Second Half of Life.* (Nashville, Discipleship Ministries, 2017.)

Moody, Harry R. and Carroll, David. *The Five Stages of the Soul.* (New York, Random House, 1999.)

Morgan, Richard L. *Remembering Your Story. Creating Your Own Spiritual Autobiography.* (Nashville, Upper Room Books, 2002.)

Nelson, John E. and Bolles, Richard N., *What Color is Your Parachute? For Retirement. Planning a Prosperous, Healthy, and Happy Future.* (Berkeley, the Speed Press, 2010.)

Osborn, Carol. *The Art of Resilience. 100 Paths to Wisdom and Strength in an Uncertain World.* (New York, Three Rivers Press, 1997.)

Peck, M. Scott. *The Road Less Travelled.* (New York, Touchstone Books, 1978.)

Pennebaker, James. *Opening Up: The Healing Power of Expressing Emotions.* (New York, the Guilford Press, 1997.)

Pinker, Susan. *The Village Effect. How Face-to-Face Contact Can Make Us Healthier and Happier.* (Toronto, Vintage Canada, 2015.)

Putnam, Robert. *Bowling Alone. The Collapse and Revival of American Community.* (New York, Simon and Schuster, 2011.)

Randolph, William B., Address at *Boomerstock*, Nashville, Tennessee. Sponsored by the United Methodist Church, September 28 to October 1, 2016.

Roberto, John. *"Faith Formation with Baby Boomers,* "in Lifelong Faith. The Theory and Practice of Lifelong Faith Formation. Volume 4.4. Winter 2010.

Robertson, Geraldine. Aamjiwnaang First Nation Elder. Interview with author, August 2016, Aamjiwnaang First Nation, Sarnia, Ontario.

Rolheiser, Ronald. *Sacred Fire. A Vision for A Deeper Human and Christian Maturity.* (New York, Image, 2014.)

Rohr, Richard. *Falling Upward. A Spiritual Journey for the Two Halves of Life.* (San Francisco, Jossey Bass, 2011.)

_____, *Healing Our Violence Through the Journey of Centring Prayer.* CD. (1705 Five Points Road SW, Albuquerque, NM 87105 Centre for Action and Contemplation, 2013.

_____, *The Art of Letting Go: Living the Wisdom of Saint Francis.* (Sounds True, CD.)

Roof, Wade Clark. *A Generation of Seekers. The Spiritual Journeys of the Baby Boom Generation.* (San Francisco, Harper, 1993.)

_____*Spiritual Marketplace: Baby Boomers and the Remaking of American Religion.* (Princeton, N.J.: Princeton University Press, 1999.)

_____and W. Carroll, and David A. Roozen, editors. *The Post-War Generation and Establishment Religion: Cross-Cultural Perspectives."* (Boulder, CO: Westview Press, 1995.)

Ross, Allen and Ross, Betty. Interview with author, July, 2016, London, Ontario.

Schachter-Shalomi, Zalman, and Miller, Ronald S. *From Age-ing to Sage-ing. A Revolutionary Approach to Growing Older.* (New York, time-Warner Books, 1997.)

Sleeth, Natalie. *"In the Bulb There is A Flower,"* hymn. Also known as Hymn of Promise, 1986 Hope Publishing Company, 380 South Main Place, Carol Stream, IL 60188 (800-323-1049)

Seligman, Martin E. P. *Authentic Happiness. Using New Positive Psychology to Realise Your Potential for Lasting Fulfillment.* (New York, The Free Press, 2002.)

_____, *Flourish. A Visionary Understanding of Happiness and Wellbeing.* (New York, The Free Press, 2011.)

Sheehy, Gail. *New Passages.* (New York, Random House, 1995.)

Smith, Walker J. and Clurman, Ann. *Rocking the Ages: The Yankelovich Report on Generational Marketing.* (New York: Harper Business, a Division of Harper Collins Publishers, 1997.)

Stevens, Rev. Matthew. Aamjiwnaang First Nation Elder. E-mail Correspondence with author, Summer 2016.

Stevens, R. Paul., *Aging Matters. Finding your calling for the rest of your life.* (Grand Rapids, William B. Eerdmann's Publishing House, 2016.)

_____Interview with author. Regent College, Vancouver, B.C., October 25, 2016, and workshop on October 29, 2016, Carey Theological College, Vancouver, B. C.

Stiegelbauer, S. M. *"What is an Elder? What do Elders Do? First nation Elders as Teachers in Culture-Based Urban organizations,"* Ontario Institute for Studies in Education of the University of Toronto.

Swinton, John, *Resurrecting the Person. Friendship and the Care of People with Mental Health Problems.* (Nashville, Abingdon Press, 2000.)

_____, *Spirituality and Mental Health Care. Rediscovering a 'Forgotten' Dimension.* (London, Jessica Kingsley Publishers, 2001.)

The United Church of Canada. *A New Creed.* 1995.

_____. *A Song of Faith.* A Statement of Faith of the United Church of Canada, L'Eglise Unie du Canada, 2006.

Thomas, Lewis H., editor. *The Making of a Socialist: The Recollections of T.C. Douglas.* (Edmonton: University of Alberta Press, 1982.)

Tindal, Mardi. *Soul Maps. A Guide to the Mid-life Spirit* (Toronto, United Church Publishing House, 2000).

Toynbee, Arnold. *A Study of History. Abridgement of Volumes 1-6.* (Oxford, Oxford University Press, 1974.)

Untermeyer, Louis. *Robert Frost's Poems.* (New York, Pocket Books, 1970.) Especially "Two Tramps in Mudtime," pp. 112-114.

Vaillant, George E. *Aging Well. Surprising Guideposts to a Happier Life from the landmark Harvard Study of Adult Development.* (New York, Hachette Book Group, 2002) E-book edition.

_____. *Triumphs of Experience. The Men of the Harvard Grant Study.* (Cambridge. The Belknapp Press of Harvard University Press, 2012.)

Veith, Gene Edward, Jr., *God at Work.* (Wheaton, Illinois, Cressway, 2002.)

Wallis, Velma. *Two Old Women: An Alaska Legend of Betrayal, Courage, and Survival.* (New York, Harper Collins, 1993.)

Walsh, Pamela, "Marcus Buckingham: Your Strengths & What Gives You Energy" in Blog: *Potential Within: Reflective Writing through Yoga. Balancing Effort and Ease on and off the Mat.* July 12, 2008.

Wingren, Gustaf. *Luther on Vocation*, Carl C. Ramussen, Trans. (Eugene, Oregon, Wipf & Stock, 2004.)

Wuthnow, Robert. *America and the Challenges of Religious Diversity.* (Princeton, Princeton University Press, 2005.)

Video Resources

Amour. Michael Haneke, Director, 2012.

Dench, Judi, Nighy, Bill, Wilkinson, Tom, Smith, Maggie. *The Best Exotic Marigold Hotel.* DVD, Directed by John Madden, 20th Century Fox, 2012.

Hope Springs. David Frankel, Director, 2012.

Nicholson, Jack. *About Schmidt.* DVD, directed by Alexander Payne, Alliance Atlantis, Montreal, 2010.

Jones, De Witt. *"For the Love of It,"* DVD. Star Thrower.

Rain Man, Film. Barry Levinson, director, 1988.

Re-Designing Your Life: A Practical Spirituality for the Second Half of Life, Sheila Macgregor. Wib Dawson, videographer and editor, 2017.

Room, Film Director: Lenny Abrahamson, 2015.

Quartet, Film, Dustin Hoffman, director. Headline Pictures, BBC Films. DCM Productions, 2012.

Acknowledgements

I am very grateful to the many who have accompanied me on this journey into the second half of life and who have supported or encouraged me in my research:

The United Church of Canada Foundation, for their generous support of my research by awarding me the McGeachy Senior Scholarship;

My wonderful congregation, Siloam United Church, London, Ontario, including my Doctor of Ministry Advisory Group: Marlene Brown, Cora Burns, Richard Cook, Wib Dawson, Anne Donkervoort, Catherine Glover, Steven Lord, and Al Newton; former Dean of the Doctor of Ministry Degree program at McCormick Theological Seminary, Jeff Japinga, who, together with my peers Tom Bryson, Cheryle Hanna, and Paula Sanders, encouraged me to make this resource available to others; my D. Min. Supervisor, Anna Case-Winters; the 24 men and women who participated in the pilot project for this program; our Administrative Assistant Erin Salter, who used her personal time to assist with some of the more technical aspects of this project; the members of the Siloam Ministry and Personnel Committee and Church Council for granting me extra time in the summer of 2016 to carry out my research and writing; and David Dillon, Marlee Chamberlain, Stuart Cunningham, and Richard

Graham, who stepped in to lead our church study groups so that I could have more time for my research;

The many people who allowed me to interview them and who shared their personal stories of the second half of life: Al Appleby, Anne Beattie-Stokes, Fran Boone, Christina Boyd, Bill and Karen Butt, Janet Christensen, Richard Cook, Susan Galbraith, Jane Kuepfer, Neil and Linda Lackey, Gary Mallalieu, Susan and David McKane, Marianne Mellinger, Joyce Payne, Vic and Helena Phillips, Jill Pillon, Elizabeth Rickerby, Geraldine Robertson, Allen and Betty Ross, Kerry Stover, and Gillian Thomas; as well as Bruce Dawson and Mike Ashton, who assisted with the set-up for some of these interviews, and Beth Roberts, who helped with their transcription;

The many individuals who read a first draft and offered their encouragement for my work: Kathy Gaskin, Jane Kuepfer, Richard Macgregor, Brad Morrison, Patricia Nicholl, Paul Pearce, and Mardi Tindal. I also greatly appreciate the helpful feedback, constructive criticisms and suggestions I received from: Anne Beattie-Stokes, Janet Christensen, Martin Ferguson, Jeff Japinga, Deborah Kapp, Alexandra Macgregor-Amde, Barbara McGill, and Will Randolph. (It goes without saying that all remaining flaws are my own!);

Rev. Wib Dawson, for so generously giving of his wisdom, time, and talents to film and edit the numerous video interviews we conducted over many weeks and months. A true renaissance man, Wib is the perfect model of one who has found deep meaning and purpose in the second half of life, as he continues to learn and grow and find new ways to respond to Christ's call. Wib's ministry and mentorship have blessed my life in countless ways over the past thirty years and I am grateful for the friendship and support he and his wife, Carol, have always given my family and me;

My children—my wonderful sons Lachlan, John, and Malcolm, for their love and patience; and of course, their big sister Alexandra for not only reading and critiquing my manuscript at various stages but especially for her unfailing support and faith in me. Every mother should be blessed by such a daughter;

Last but far from least, my loving and devoted husband and best friend, Richard, who has brought me more joy than I could ever have imagined in the first half of life and with whom I share a marvellous second half! I pray that we may enjoy many more happy years together as we continue to navigate the afternoon of life.

Sheila Macdonald Macgregor,
January 1st, 2018,
Exeter, Ontario

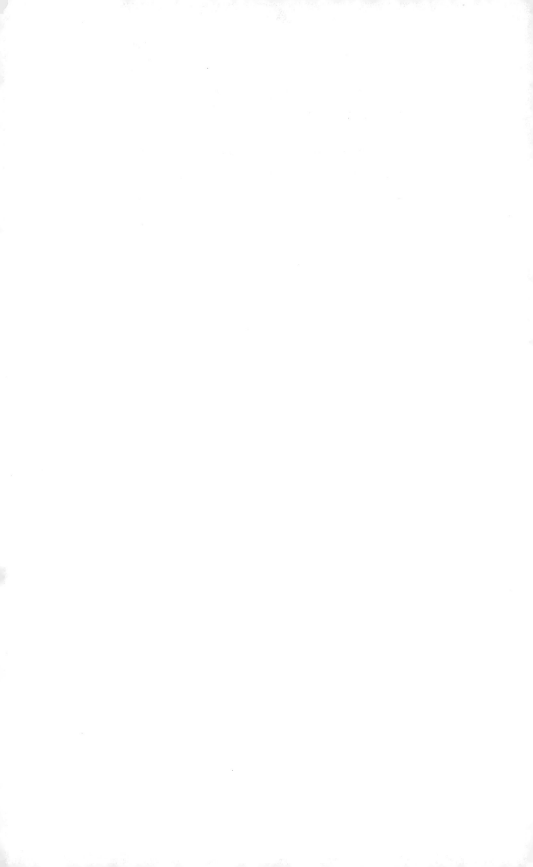

CPSIA information can be obtained
at www.ICGtesting.com
Printed in the USA
LVHW04s0032260618
581875LV00001B/1/P